GLOBAL FLUIDS

Fertility, Reproduction and Sexuality

For a full volume listing please see back matter.

GLOBAL FLUIDS

The Cultural Politics of Reproductive Waste and Value

Charlotte Kroløkke

berghahn
NEW YORK • OXFORD
www.berghahnbooks.com

First published in 2018 by
Berghahn Books
www.berghahnbooks.com

Library of Congress Cataloging-in-Publication Data

Names: Kroløkke, Charlotte, author.
Title: Global fluids: The Cultural Politics of Reproductive Waste and Value / Charlotte Kroløkke.
Description: New York: Berghahn Books, 2018 | Series: Fertility, Reproduction and Sexuality; 39 | Includes bibliographical references and index.
Identifiers: LCCN 2018015958 (print) | LCCN 2018023952 (ebook) | ISBN 9781785338939 (eBook) | ISBN 9781785338922 (hardback: alk. paper)
Subjects: LCSH: Human reproductive technology. | Human reproduction.
Classification: LCC RG133.5 (ebook) | LCC RG133.5 .K76 2018 (print) | DDC 618.1/7806--dc23
LC record available at https://lccn.loc.gov/2018015958

British Library Cataloguing in Publication Data

A catalogue record for this book is available from the British Library.

ISBN 978-1-78533-892-2 hardback
ISBN 978-1-78533-893-9 ebook

To Theo and Valentin
for their laughter and love

Contents

List of Figures and Illustrations viii

Acknowledgments ix

Introduction 1

Chapter 1. Scholarly Conversation 21

Chapter 2. Urine: From Waste to Hormone Shots 52

Chapter 3. Oocytes: From Waste to Assets 81

Chapter 4. Placentas: From Waste to Regeneration 110

Conclusion 140

Bibliography 167

Index 183

Figures and Illustrations

Figure 0.1. Mapping empirical sites 14

Figure 1.1. Oocytes as global fluids 46

Figure 1.2. Placenta as global fluid 48

Figure 1.3. Urine as global fluid 49

Figure 2.1. Pregnyl 57

Figure 2.2. Menopur 57

Figure 2.3. Early urine collection 58

Figure 2.4. Urine collection 58

Figure 2.5. Urine collection set 58

Figure 4.1. Lotus birth 114

Figure 4.2. Mother and son 114

Figure 4.3. Mother, grandmother, and son 114

Figure 4.4. Placenta 116

Figure 4.5. Trash 116

Figure 4.6. Container 116

Figure 4.7. Placenta encapsulation 121

Figure 4.8. Dried umbilical cord 121

Figure 4.9. Japan Bio Products 124

Figure 5.1. The altruism/commodification logics 142

Acknowledgments

This book owes a great deal to many colleagues, friends, students, and family members. Thank you to the University of Southern Denmark for funding the research project Reproductive Medicine and Mobility (REMM) and to the group of fun REMM colleagues: Karen Hvidtfeldt Madsen, Matilde Lykkebo Petersen, Frank Høgholm Pedersen, Kent Kristensen, Tine Tjørnhøj-Thomsen, Jens Fedder, and Michael Nebeling Petersen. I am grateful that several of you volunteered to read and comment on earlier drafts: thank you Michael Nebeling for always providing inspirational comments, and thank you Dag Heede for your generosity and sharp analytical skills that always push me to improve my work.

Institutional support and funding agencies have made my research and writing easier: Thank you to Anne Jensen for your administrative support, and to Marianne Lysholt, Lene Vivi Petersen, and Dorte Winther for assistance in administering my, at times, impressive amount of travel receipts. Thank you also to the Danish Research Council, which twice supported my study.

An inspiring and wonderful group of collaborators has been crucial throughout: Thank you to Karen A. Foss and Elizabeth Dickinson, whose work on placentas as forms of communication was pivotal to me. Thank you Stine Willum Adrian, Janne Rothmar Herrmann, Katherine Carroll, Jette Rygaard, Filareti Kotsi, Catherine Waldby, Yael Hashiloni-Dolev, Kinneret Lahad, Ayo Wahlberg, Lene Myong, Hiromi Tanaka, Minori Kokado, Nicky Hudson, Lorraine Culley, Kathrin Maurer, and Chia-Ling Wu for your encouragements and ideas. Thank you also to the clinical collaborators Yael Kramer, David Keefe, Lucy Lu, David McCulloh, Cristina Pozzobon, Jurie van den Elsen—without your support and openness this research would not have been possible. Thank you to wonderful research assistants:

Anne Vestergaard Yousufi, Hanne Poulsen, and Lone Sommer, and thank you to Marcia Inhorn who continues to impress and inspire.

A very special thank you to my sister whose strength and insight I greatly admire, and to the Five College Women's Studies Research Center, including Nayiree Roubinian and Jennifer Hamilton, who so generously granted me a research stay at Mount Holyoke College during which I completed my work.

And last but certainly not least, thank you to Michael Warnock, whose patience and understanding has been invaluable, and to our sons Theo and Valentin, whose presence always reminds me of what really matters. This book is for you!

INTRODUCTION

The body has become a goldmine of usable parts (Jones 2016). In the United States, a woman may earn $20,000 to $35,000 as a surrogate; a sperm provider will receive in the range of $35 to $200 for his gametes, while egg donation ranges between $5,000 and $10,000 (Jones 2016). Other bodily parts are usable as well: hair can be sold (price depends on color, thickness, length, and ethnicity of donor, but generally ranges between $100 and $4,000 at Hairwork.com); blood plasma obtains $20 to $60 per donation (Morgan 2016); breast milk grants the producer between $300 and $1,200 for a month's supply when disseminated through the organization onlythebreast.com;[1] stool can now be provided to the organization OpenBiome, which redistributes it to help treat individuals suffering from gastrointestinal distress (annual compensation of approximately $13,000) (Alter 2016; Morgan 2016); whole bodies can temporarily be donated to NASA, who will pay $18,000 if the provider is willing to lie in bed for 70 days (Morgan 2016), while a single cadaver may generate between $110,000 and $222,000 in potential fees and revenue (Parry 2007: 1138). What may be considered bodily waste, usable parts, vacant bodies, or simply extractable material has contributed to an emerging relationship between the body and commerce, fueled by scientific and technological progress and developments.

This book is about the ways that pregnant women's urine, placentas, and oocytes become exchangeable. Women's reproductive donations gain (new) meaning throughout their extraction, industrialization, commodification, and consumption processes. I begin the book by outlining and developing a feminist cultural analytical approach to reproductive donations, and I conclude it by extending the analyses of reproductive donations to feminist bioethics and cultural politics. What, I ask, happens to our understanding of urine, oocytes, and placentas when they circulate and become exchangeable? For example, how does a temporary reproductive organ such as the placenta move from being understood as waste, biohazard material, or baby's first home to turn up again as a central ingredient in a smoothie, as medicine, and in anti-aging, whitening cream? What is the trajectory that enables pregnant women's urine, commonly framed as waste (best to be avoided, forgotten, and promptly flushed), to be donated and turned into fertility hormones and pregnancy kits? Similarly, how do oocytes through communication, clinical, and cultural practices move from being inside one woman to being extracted, cryopreserved, fertilized, and seen as "naturally" belonging to another? And what are the moral limits involved that would dictate what reproductive matter or fluids can move into the global marketplace?

Throughout the book, the idea of "global fluids" works as an analytical device. It brings to the foreground how reproductive matter, in more ways than one, has obtained global and liquid qualities. Notably, while oocytes and urine are fluids to some extent, the placenta is an organ. Attached to the lining of the womb, the placenta manages nutrients to the baby and serves as a waste disposer of sorts. So the concept of global fluids does not refer only to the liquid qualities of a particular reproductive donation. More importantly, it makes reference to the fact that reproductive donations have become liquid and globalized, along with cultural values, laws, exchange systems, and ethics. Hence, I stress the need to understand biological matter as material flows rather than merely physical entities (Hoeyer 2013), and, in a similar way as Morse (1990: 194), I note that liquidity refers to "the exchange of values between different ontological levels and otherwise incommensurable facets of life." From an economic point of view, women's reproductive donations may also be liquid in the sense that they are easy to exchange and convert into profit. So the notions of "global" and "fluids" become metaphors for the ways that reproductive matter, cultural values, laws, money, and ethics travel and move across national and cultural borders and imaginaries, situating the idea of "global" as a "discursive condition" and a cultural imaginary more than as an actual reality (Franklin et al. 2000: 4).

Global Fluids is embedded in feminist, sociological, and anthropological scholarship, and the scholarship of science and technology studies, and so extends the existing scholarship on reproductive donations into new empirical domains (Almeling 2011; Dickenson 2009; Inhorn 2015; Kroløkke 2009; Mamo 2007; Melhuus 2012;

Roberts 2012; Scheper-Hughes 2001, 2005; Sharp 2000; Thompson 2005). While feminist scholarship has already placed gender in the foreground in the analyses of reproductive donations (Almeling 2011; Daniels 2006; Konrad 2005, 2000; Nahman 2011, 2013; Roberts 2012), little research has centered on the work that goes into urine or placenta donation. In fact, feminist cultural analyses of urine donation are missing entirely, while analyses of placenta donations are rare (exceptions include Passariello 1994; Kroløkke et al. 2016; Dickinson et al. 2016). Similarly, while feminist scholars have tended to focus on the experiences of patients, and to a lesser extent on gamete providers and surrogates, they still need to turn their analyses to the emergent markets in in vitro fertilization (IVF) instruments, reagents, technologies, and cryopreservation media, for example. The scholarly attention that some body parts or some reproductive entities and relations are given is not only a facet of their reproductive role but is also intertwined with the cultural values in which reproductive parts and social relations are embedded, including the fact that while some body parts remain inside the body (such as oocytes), other parts are expelled from it and more readily enter into a waste and exchange economy (such as urine and placentas).

Throughout the book I discuss the ways that reproduction is entangled with neoliberal ideology. A central argument is the notion that neoliberal discourses not only facilitate that reproductive donations are moved from the arena of reproductive waste to reproductive value, but they also make this move appear legitimate, even natural. I position neoliberalism as a "set of dispersed discourses, positions and practices inflected by the specificity of the different contexts in which it emerges" (Walkerdine and Bansel 2010: 492). Within neoliberal ideology, individuals are cast as responsible for their fertility and for making behavioral choices that maximize their chances of pregnancy and upward mobility (Kroløkke and Pant 2012). Under this framework, reproductive matter is turned into particular types of commodities and reproduction becomes privatized, available for investment and speculation. Because neoliberal discourses put a premium on the construction of active, responsible, and positive (reproductive) actors (Newman et al. 2007), the providers of these reproductive donations—whether it be oocyte, urine, or placenta providers—are most often positioned as active and rational choice-making individuals. As noted by Rose (1999), neoliberal ideology produces individuals who become entrepreneurs of themselves, capable of transforming their lives to optimize and enhance their life circumstances.

In the arena of reproductive donations, neoliberal discourses are frequently supplemented with the more sanctioned discourse of the gift (Gunnarson and Svenaeus 2012; Kroløkke 2014). This is readily seen when the money that egg providers receive is positioned as "compensation" rather than "payment." It is taken out of the monetary realm and narrated instead as altruism combined with a desire to give someone else the gift of motherhood (Almeling 2011; Parry 2007; Pollock 2003; Roberts 2012). To Parry (2007: 1140), the use of the compensation discourse is a cover-up for a "collective squeamishness" associated with money changing hands between different and differently positioned reproductive actors. The way that the preferred scheme of neoliberal gifting operates is also seen in the choice to position the women and men who participate in this emergent market rhetorically as "donors" rather than as "workers," "sellers," or, the term used throughout this book, "providers." Clearly when gift-giving becomes the preferred metaphor, it has the effect of positioning reproductive provider bodies as legitimately constructed for someone else's desire and needs (Pollock 2003; Raymond 1993). Because altruism draws upon cultural notions of dignity and integrity, reproduction gets repositioned in the private, intimate sphere of an individual woman who intends to become a mother and individual women who desire to help other women through providing them with their eggs or urine, rather than larger economic and resource market–like forces. This is reinstated in the clinical setting when the fertilized provider egg, during the embryo implantation procedure, is positioned as having no ties to the woman it came from but instead carries the recipient woman's name on the petri dish. It is similarly present in the latest Swedish and Danish debates on uterine transplants, in which a known living donor (frequently the woman's mother, a sibling, or a friend) donates her uterus to help a known recipient (daughter, sister, or friend) experience pregnancy and birth (Kroløkke and Nebeling 2017). In the latter case, a complicated transplant procedure is positioned as a legitimate donation (unlike a commercial surrogacy arrangement), granting the recipient woman her "natural" and "legitimate" desire not only for a child but also the experience involved in pregnancy and birth, making the uterus a shared object of desire, effectively turning the vacant uterus into an exchangeable entity and reinstating the idea that birthing is a prerequisite of motherhood (Kroløkke and Nebeling 2017).

In this book I view the reproductive body as a resource within an emergent and globalized tissue economy that seeks to optimize the reproductive body's potential (Gunnarson and Svenaeus 2012; Rose 2007; Waldby and Mitchell 2006). To Rose, technological developments are not only "merely a triumph of surgical technique" but should also be seen within concerted efforts that are "oriented towards the goal of optimization" (Rose 2007: 17). Rose (2007) notes that optimization has a moral imperative. This is readily seen, for example, in cases of women who electively choose to freeze their eggs and take on the position of the responsible reproductive citizen, acting upon anticipations associated with their potential future, (failed) fertility (Carroll and Kroløkke 2017; van de Wiel 2015; Waldby 2014). It is similarly the case when pregnant women's urine gains new value through industrial (maximization) processes or when animal placentas are collected by the Danish pig farmers, placed into plastic bags, rushed to the freezers, picked up in company vans for further processing, and sent to the Asian pharmaceutical and cosmetics industry, constituting new ways for the Danish pig farmers to turn reproductive "waste" into profits.

Reproductive donations are increasingly entangled with a transnational market in reproduction. This is evident in chapter 3, for example, when I turn to the European exchanges in oocytes. The oocyte economy is increasingly predicated on a mix of recipients who are willing to travel transnationally for treatment, egg providers who are similarly willing to travel to provide clinics (and other women) with their genetic material, and vitrification technologies sophisticated enough to enable oocytes to be stored and shipped transnationally. In this manner, recipients, providers, and reproductive matter are on the move. As far as patients or recipients are concerned, Shenfield et al. (2010) point to a minimum of twenty-four to thirty thousand cycles of cross-border fertility treatments that could be taking place each year throughout Europe, involving as many as eleven thousand to fourteen thousand patients. While research within the social sciences has tended to prioritize the recipient (couples), much less is known about women who travel transnationally to provide other women with their oocytes. Nevertheless, agencies such as Global Egg Donors (United States) and Traveling Donors (South Africa) specialize in "global donors" (Kroløkke 2016a, 2015). Similarly, only few scholars have centered the multiple relations that unfold when vitrified eggs travel across borders (exceptions include Nahman 2013). In these transnational encounters, oocytes gain potential and value in the narratives of recipients, clinicians, and providers alike (Kroløkke 2016a, 2015).

Reproductive donations such as urine and placenta are similarly vital ingredients in the emergent international pharmaceutical and cosmetics industry. With an estimated $1.5 billion in the United States alone, the IVF-related pharmaceutical industry is big business. In the specific case of fertility hormones, women's urine is used as an ingredient in the development of products such as Pregnyl and Menopur, developed by large international pharmaceutical companies and sold to women worldwide. Considered a natural protein hormone, Pregnyl is administered, for example, in IVF treatments (including to women going through IVF, as well as to egg providers, of course) and it is frequently known as the trigger shot used to bring on ovulation during IVF. Additionally, male athletes can use Pregnyl as a testosterone booster, while there are a few reports of it reportedly having been prescribed by medical doctors as a slimming drug.[2] In comparison, human and animal placentas enter the European as well as Asian pharmaceutical and cosmetics industries. For example, Japan Bio Products has more than forty years of experience using human and animal placental extract in the development of pharmaceutical and cosmetics products, selling its products throughout Asia. Founded in Japan, the company is now situated in Taiwan, Korea, China, Hong Kong, Vietnam, the United States, and Switzerland.[3]

Potentiality is a prerequisite in the circulation of reproductive waste. As a concept, it refers to the personal, commercial, and/or biomedical benefits that, in this case, reproductive donations hold. According to Taussig et al., potentiality situates bodily matter as plastic—capable of being transmuted "into something completely different" (Taussig et al. 2013: S4). Rhetorically framed as "power," "potens," and "force," the concept of potentiality suggests that biological matter is adaptable and open to human modification (Taussig et al. 2013: S4). In the case of a reproductive organ, such as the human placenta, it moves from being a "life generator" and "protector" to having no future potential—being scrutinized for its appearance and transferred following the afterbirth for further testing or to the garbage bin. However, the placenta obtains new potentiality as a postpartum preventative measure, energizer, and whitening or anti-aging lotion, through human and industrial modification. Similarly, women's urine moves from having no potential or force to becoming a valuable ingredient in the development of fertility drugs, through industrial and commercial undertakings. Even the egg provider's genetic material is frequently positioned as "wasted" matter—not used by the provider herself and thus open for being entered into a "gifting" economy, in which the provider engages in the altruistic act of helping someone else achieve motherhood.

Feminist and consumer study scholars add important theoretical frameworks to critically understand the workings of potentiality. For example, Morgan (2013) points out how potentiality is gendered and embedded in moral reasoning. In the specific case of abortion debates in the United States, she argues that the choice to view the developing fetus in its early stages as a potential future citizen or human being paradoxically takes place "at the expense of the potential for pregnant women to exercise their own interpretations of liberty and choice" (Morgan 2013: S17). Moreover, the ways in which female bodily emissions, such as menstruation, are framed as sources of impurity or bodily waste—fluids with no potential—is predicated on a gendered hierarchy (Martin 2001; Shail 2007). Similarly, the interplay between the inside and the outside of the body is another type of gendered ordering, in which women's reproductive emissions (such as menstruation, placentas, and breast milk) get de- and revalued (Douglas [1966] 1984). This is in sharp contrast to men's bodily emissions, such as Danish sperm, which have readily entered the global bioeconomy as a valuable export commodity (Kroløkke 2009; Martin 1991).

This book is built upon an interdisciplinary and theoretical mix of feminist, sociological, anthropological, and science and technology scholarship theorizing the ways that women's reproductive donations, exemplified in the three case studies of eggs, urine, and placentas, gain new value and take on new biographies. The choice to center eggs, urine, and placentas is done to show how different parts of women's reproductive bodies are differently mobilized. Obviously, urine, eggs, and placentas are all fluids or reproductive matter derived from women's reproductive labor, yet the ways in which they circulate differ tremendously. Instead of acting as representative categories, however, women's reproductive fluids serve as "indicative instances" or "orienteering devices" (Franklin et al. 2000: 11) that open up a more general discussion of the gendering of the contemporary repro-economy. While I return to the theoretical framework, including a feminist cultural analytical perspective in chapter 1 and the feminist cultural politics on reproductive donations in my conclusion, I now briefly touch upon the methodological approaches undertaken, including my use of the concept of *assemblage ethnography,* in order to define the work that goes into this book.

Assemblage Ethnography: Analytical and Empirical Tracking Strategies

In *Global Fluids* I develop three case studies and combine a diverse set of empirical data. I suggest the term *assemblage ethnography* to help frame the analytical and empirical methodologies that may go into this feminist cultural analytical research.[4] In my use of the term, it embraces the use of diverse empirical material, from legal and ethical guidelines, governmental debates, interview transcripts, and ethnographic fieldwork on various sites to popular media accounts, literary texts, health campaigns, advertisements, online discussion groups, and expert interviews. As such, and as it is used in this book, assemblage ethnography bears a resemblance to the concept of multi-sited ethnography developed by Marcus (1999). The ambition to use a new methodological vocabulary, however, is similar to Roberts's (2015) coining of bio-ethnography as a way to capture her biological and ethnographic data. Whereas feminist cultural analysis historically has relied upon a wealth of methods derived from the social sciences as well as the humanities, the choice to center the assemblage concept, in this case, highlights ties to queer studies, sociological and anthropological work, as well as the diverse empirical material that goes into *Global Fluids*.

In my use of the term, assemblage ethnography suggests an analytical as well as an empirical tracking strategy. Analytically, assemblage thinking has gained currency in queer and literary studies (Puar 2007), as well as in sociological and anthropological work (Ong and Collier 2005 Marcus and Saka 2006; Rose 2007). It has become a framework for conceptualizing "shifting relations and emergent conditions of spatially distributed objects of study" (Marcus and Saka 2006: 106). For example, Ong and Collier (2005) use the notion of assemblage to critically examine how globalization and neoliberalism come together along lines of gender, sexuality, and neocolonialism, whereas Puar (2007) employs assemblage thinking to show how nationality, sexuality, gender, ethnicity, and class entangle. Within the realm of feminist and queer scholarship on reproduction, Nebeling et al. (2016) use the concept to show how affects and discourses on surrogacy in Norwegian media debates mix to reinstate the Norwegian nation-state as exceptional and superior. Similarly, Kroløkke (2016b) illustrates how "IVF holidays" in Barbados are assembled through affects of hope and neocolonial fantasies of the tropical island. Jointly, these scholars note that assemblage thinking is best understood as "an evocation of emergence and heterogeneity" (Marcus and Saka 2006: 106), or perhaps even as a verb (Holliday et al. 2015).

So what is added in taking an assemblage empirical approach to the reproductive donations of eggs, urine, and placentas? First, assemblage thinking has primarily been used either as an overall theoretical frame or as an analytical tool.[5] To prioritize assemblage thinking as an analytical as well as an empirical tracking device means recognizing the multiple and heterogeneous ways that reproductive donations come to be enacted in discursive, affective, technological, and situated practices, as well as how they frequently entangle. It involves understanding the making of waste and value as dynamic and relational processes. Lury captures this when she notes that assemblages are both spaces to be mapped as well as temporal moments—they are "spatio-temporalized" (Lury 2011: 75). Akin to this, Hawkins (2011) shows how both material and discursive entanglements, in the specific case of bottled water, come to matter in different assemblages—from the branding and selling of bottled water to campaigns involving the recycling of bottles and the decision to not use bottles. While the material presence of the bottle in Hawkins's (2011) analysis is placed in the foreground, the different assemblages are distinctly political, in the sense that they speak to questions of practice and the role of the discursive material within it. As an analytical and methodological device, assemblages illustrate the ways that people, things, technologies, media, and texts interrelate (Bennett and Healy 2009).

Practically, assemblage ethnography in this book involves the collection of a diverse set of empirical material as well as the examination of different sites of study. It includes work undertaken during a five-year period from 2011 to 2016, ranging from interviews with different reproductive actors—such as patients traveling from Denmark to Spain for egg donation; clinical directors in Denmark, the United States, and Spain; international fertility clinic coordinators in Spain; marketing CEOs of pharmaceutical and cosmetics companies in Japan and the Netherlands—to field observations undertaken at select fertility clinics, along with an archive of egg-provider stories and different documents in context (marketing material, webpages, legal briefs, financial statements, online urine provider stories and images, for example). Whereas interviewing and field observations are well-suited for getting in-depth knowledge about experiences and concerns, as well as an understanding of the storytelling that takes place in social interactions (whether with donors, clinicians, lawmakers, or ethicists), documents in context, such as legal briefs or clinical webpages, add an important piece to the overall understanding of the cultural context, the practices and the communication that take place among key stakeholders, including the ways in which donors, destinations, or bodily fluids become constructed as (un)desirable.

In each case study, I unfold how a particular reproductive fluid comes into existence in an assemblage of images, commercials, texts, field observations, interviews, photos, and public and ethical debates. At times, the selection of empirical material is characterized by what Thompson calls "an excess of data" (Thompson 2013: 12). This is notably the case with the chapter on oocytes (chapter 3), in which, in an environment of fluctuating donation laws, changing yet always heated ethical debates, different compensation practices, emergent clinics, and the increasing normalization of freezing technologies, I had to prioritize certain kinds of sites, reproductive actors, and documents. In contrast, a very different assemblage emerges from the case studies on urine (chapter 2) and placentas (chapter 4). In these two cases, hesitant gatekeepers and language barriers (Dutch and Japanese) are combined with some, albeit not an overwhelming amount of, national debates. In combination, access to urine and placenta sites and stories was much more difficult and cumbersome. Consequently, each case chapter will reveal how a reproductive donation, in a very specific localized context and within a very specific set of empirical data, comes to matter and at times transfers into a global icon or traverses national borders.

While the choice to center urine, eggs, and placentas is not done with the specific aim of theorizing the ways that these fluids or matter come together, nor is the collection of diverse empirical work used to validate particular research findings. Quite to the contrary, I wish to illustrate how global fluids circulate and take on different meanings for the different reproductive actors involved, while unfolding in different cultural contexts. As noted by Thompson, in her use of "triage" as a methodological tool, urgency is a pivotal marker used to select and foreground certain types of data (Thompson 2013: 12). *Global Fluids* builds upon this notion of urgency in turning to key international sites yet notably prioritizing European sites and stories. According to Lie and Lykke (2017), turning empirically to European and non-English-speaking geographical areas enables different issues and questions to come to the fore. Consequently, while the United Kingdom, the United States, and Japan are interesting as far as placenta consumption and egg freezing is concerned, I rely more heavily on empirical material from Denmark, Spain, and the

Netherlands to illustrate the ways that oocytes, placentas, and urine flow. A brief introduction to these sites and their importance is, accordingly, in order.

Briefly, Denmark is an especially interesting case study. A fertility destination for single and lesbian women, Denmark is additionally a point of departure for intending families in need of oocytes or surrogacy (Adrian and Kroløkke 2018) as well as a vital exporter of reproductive tissue such as bull sperm (reappearing as Viking genetics) and porcine placentas (now staged as "organic Danish pigs") to the Asian agricultural, pharmaceutical, and cosmetics industry. Of particular importance in the Danish IVF assemblage is the law on assisted reproduction, which permits anonymous and known sperm donation to single women as well as lesbian couples. IVF to women older than forty-five years are banned, while a maximum oocyte freezing period of five years has made social freezing difficult at best. In combination, the Danish law has effectively led to an outflow of infertile women and couples to other European countries, notably Spain. While the Danish compensation for oocytes has changed dramatically in the recent years, during the research period of 2011–2016, compensation was low (ranging between eighty and three hundred euros), resulting in a significant shortage of oocyte providers.

The Danish version of the welfare state is key to understanding contemporary Danish biopolitics on assisted reproductive technologies. Not only is reproduction and IVF state sanctioned, the making of children is also encouraged and seen as a state matter, and as essential in the continuation of the Danish welfare state. This understanding has resulted in generous family leave policies as well as free access to medically assisted reproduction to women who do not already have children (and are under forty years of age at the point of referral) or to lesbian and heterosexual couples who do not already have one joint child. Once the child is born, the Danish state grants all parents child support, and children have access to free public education, healthcare, and vaccinations, while daycare centers are, in the case of lower-income or single parents, made available at a reduced price. To Melhuus (2012), the Nordic welfare states entangle with Lutheran principles on equality and welfare centering what has come to be known as "family values." Meanwhile, not all ways of becoming a family or all types of families are state sanctioned or viewed as morally just (Melhuus 2012). In the Danish version of the welfare state, this is evident when the desire to have at least one joint child (as in the case of the aforementioned couples receiving free IVF) is naturalized as at the core of the Danish nuclear family. It is similarly present in the contemporary Danish debates potentially granting child support to a maximum of three children. Here, it simultaneously becomes a way of managing what is seen as the immigrant population's "uncontrolled fertility." Thus, the Danish biopolitics on reproduction advances the making of not only children but also particular types of (Danish) families and parents.

While Denmark has established itself as a European hub for anonymous and known sperm donation, during the 2011–16 period, women over the age of forty-five (who in the Danish context could not legally receive IVF) as well as women (and couples) in need of oocyte donation (and no longer willing or able to remain on the Danish waiting lists) traveled out of Denmark to other European locales. In this context, Spain emerged as a popular reproductive hub. The Spanish clinics have successfully branded themselves as quality clinics characterized by high success rates, a multilingual group of fertility doctors (frequently matching the international patients with a similar-language doctor), customer-oriented coordinators, well-developed clinical websites, relations with select Danish clinics along with the availability of a wide range of oocyte providers (due to the compensation of approximately one thousand euros), and an ability (as well as requirement) to match phenotypes (race, eye, and hair color in particular) of the providers with that of the recipients. Orobitg and Salazar (2005) locate the Spanish success story within a liberal law and a history of noninterventionist policies, turning reproduction and the making of families into a private affair. Consequently, egg donation is legal and all donations are anonymous, donations must be carried out in authorized centers, providers are compensated, and clinics are required to match the phenotypes of recipients with those of the providers. Similarly, in an ethnographic study of German women traveling to Spain and the Czech Republic for egg donation, Bergmann notes how the entanglements of an existing tourism infrastructure, international airports, and business amenities have turned cities like Barcelona and Prague into "global cities" of reproduction (Bergmann 2011: 601).

Meanwhile, the donation of urine has a long history of being organized and undertaken in the Netherlands. The Dutch story is, in several ways, unique. In the Netherlands, pharmaceutical companies had yet to be created during the early 1920s, and the development of the first pharmaceutical company emerged out of the joint efforts of Ernst Laqueur (head of the leading Dutch research group in endocrinology) and Saal van Zwanenberg (owner of a slaughterhouse located in Oss, the Netherlands) (Oudshoorn 1994). While van Zwanenberg wanted to manage organic waste, Laqueur sought to secure a steady supply of research material (Oudshoorn 1994). As a result of this collaboration, the pharmaceutical company Organon Limited Company was founded in 1923 (Oudshoorn 1994). While its first product was insulin, Organon began to produce estrogen in the 1930s. When German scientists discovered that pregnant women's urine was high in hormones, the production of estrogen became entangled during this time period with this new raw material. Consequently, Organon, along with other European pharmaceutical companies, extended their relations to gynecologists who could acquire women's urine during their prenatal visits (Oudshoorn 1994). Later in the 1930s when these European scientists discovered that pregnant mares could provide an even larger amount of hormone-rich urine, farmers became pivotal to the production of sex hormones. In the case of the Netherlands, however, the use of pregnant women's urine continued and is now organized and managed through the Dutch organization Moeders voor Moeders (Mothers for Mothers). In this manner, the Dutch story reveals—as does the European story on the pharmaceutical development of sex hormones, and as Oudshoorn (1994) shows in her history of the development of sex hormones—intimate and shifting entanglements among scientific communities (research labs), businesses (slaughterhouse and farmers), and medical entities (gynecologists).

Denmark, Spain, and the Netherlands have their own distinct nationalized stories and legislation enabling the development of particular reproductive pathways in and out of these three countries (Adrian and Kroløkke 2018). Nevertheless, within the European Union, member states must also adhere to the Convention on Human Rights and Biomedicine. According to the explanatory report to this treatise, the human body and its parts must not be bought or sold (Council of Europe 1997: § 132).[6] The convention does not inhibit providers (such as oocyte providers) in receiving compensation, however, as long as it does not "give rise to financial gain for the person from whom they have been removed or for a third party, whether an individual or a corporate entity such as, for example, a hospital" (Council of Europe 1997: § 132). Meanwhile, the explanatory report makes a clear distinction between matter which is naturally expelled from the body which is made exempt: "The provision does not refer to such products as hair and nails, which are discarded tissues, and the sale of which is not an affront to human dignity" (Council of Europe 1997: §133). Whereas women's

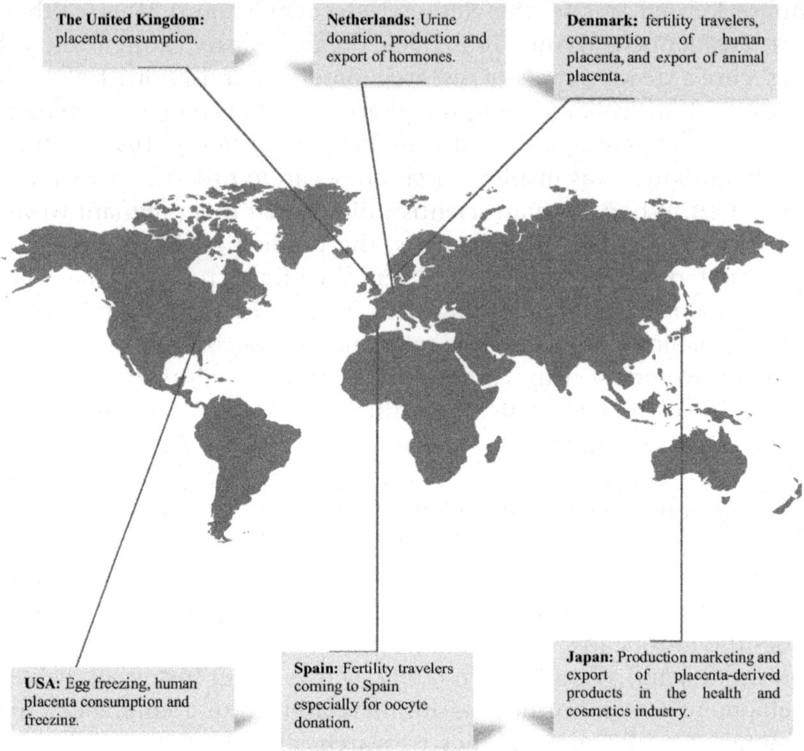

FIGURE 0.1. Mapping empirical sites: patients traveling for oocytes, urine-derived products entering the fertility industry, human placenta consumption, and animal placentas circulating to Asian pharmaceutical companies. This map is by no means a comprehensive map of how reproductive substances and organs, within Europe, move; rather, it exclusively details some of the primary sites, stories, and individuals that go into this particular set of assemblage ethnography undertaken during the time period of 2011–16. The directionality and speed with which reproductive fluids move are the products of various entanglements involving national and international legal stipulations, scientific discoveries, business and personal relations, tourism and travel infrastructures, clinical and technological expertise, as well as cultural imaginaries on who and what should be able to travel.

eggs are extracted through surgical procedures, as evidenced in this provision, urine and placentas are more readily made to appear as discarded fluids and tissue.

In *Global Fluids* I treat reproductive fluids as hybrid and very localized assemblages involving clinical expertise, instruments, persons, social relations, ideas on ownership, legal stipulations, transportation, freezers, buildings, and spaces, to name a few, involving empirical work undertaken in Spain, Denmark, Japan, and the Netherlands. This understanding entails tracking how reproductive donations take form as they are assembled and given value. In this second meaning of the term, assemblage ethnography involves understanding how reproductive donations are assembled along frequently gendered, sexualized, racialized, and nationalized values. In the case of Denmark, for example, sperm has become an export commodity, while eggs, in the first law on assisted reproduction in 1997, were not even allowed to leave the country.[7] As noted by Rose (2007), understanding the ways that reproductive donations take on different values entails the conceptualizing of these donations as more than physical matter extracted through the development of particular reproductive techniques and frequently conceptualized through commercial and economic means. Notably, such an understanding involves tracing how reproductive fluids "engender certain ways of thinking about reproduction, for the subject and for the expert, certain routines and rituals, techniques of testing and practices of fiscalization, modes of advice giving and the like" (Rose 2007: 17). When employed as an analytical device, assemblage ethnography then turns to how reproductive fluids travel. This includes how laws, ethics, practices, and stories enable traveling and entangle with discourses and affects in different empirical contexts. In the process, reproductive donations, and the cultural paths that enable these to circulate, also achieve a certain degree of liquidity.

The Structure of the Book

The book is divided into four chapters. It begins with a presentation of feminist, cultural, and analytical perspectives, including pertinent theoretical perspectives on how to study global reproductive fluids. In this first chapter, "Scholarly Conversation," I stress the need to theorize the cultural paths and routes that enable reproductive donations to move and circulate in particular ways. Throughout this chapter, reproductive donations are framed as "living things"—achieving, losing, and gaining value, enabling certain kinds of relationships, and having particular careers (Kopytoff 1986). Following the theoretical setup, I turn to three in-depth case studies on reproductive donations: urine, oocyte, and placenta donations (chapters 2–4). In the case studies, feminist cultural analyses of written documents, online marketing material, field observations, and interviews work to illustrate how a particular reproductive donation achieves value in specific entanglements. I end the book by discussing the cultural politics of reproductive waste and value, including feminist bioethical concerns on the fragmented reproductive body, and I embed this discussion in earlier arguments involving reproductive choice and agency, as well as the inadequacy of the gift/market economic framework (Shildrick 2008).

In the first case study (chapter 2), I turn to urine donation in the Netherlands, in which pregnant women donate their urine to Moeders voor Moeders. Urine is collected between the sixth and sixteenth week of pregnancy. This is the time when the hormone human chorionic gonadotropin (better known as hCG hormone) is at its highest level. To the pregnant woman, the hCG hormone helps form the placenta and contributes to the nourishment of the fertilized oocytes. When processed by the fertility company Akzo Pharma (formerly Dutch, but now owned by the South African company Aspen Pharmacare), urine is turned into a main ingredient in the development of fertility hormones and hCG pregnancy test kits. This first case study includes online donor stories, marketing material, and field studies in the Moeders voor Moeders organization and the Akzo Pharma factory in the Netherlands. My interest rests with the ways providers account and narrate their experiences, the provider recruitment efforts carried out by Moeders voor Moeders, the practices involved in exchanging urine (including pick-up and processing), and thus the ways in which urine is turned into "liquid gold."

The second case study focuses on oocyte donation (chapter 3). It illustrates how oocytes move from being understood as excess and wasteful material to becoming not only gifts but also, as evident in the Spanish case, an outgoing and loving baby. In the case of global egg providers, eggs turn into intelligent, mobile matter and, when vitrified for later use, become frozen assets. When oocytes enter the fertility industry, they acquire a biography of their own, frequently drawing upon conventional (and national) stereotypes, fantasies, and imaginations, in this case between the West and the East. In the case of Danish women traveling to Spain for treatment, reproductive matter becomes embedded in stereotypes of character and temperament, re-naturalizing national differences while also mobilizing a tale of "exotic" likeness between donors and recipients. The case study is based on interviews with Danish fertility travelers, Danish and Spanish clinical directors, marketing material, and also clinical observations in a leading Spanish fertility clinic. To discuss the ways in which eggs become not only mobile, globalized fluids but also "frozen assets," I turn to interviews with elective freezers in New York City and include a sensory ethnographic approach to a "take back your fertility" seminar on elective freezing in London.

In the final case study (chapter 4), I analyze how human and animal placentas move from being byproducts of birth or reproductive waste to becoming medicine, anti-aging, and beautifying ingredients in East Asian and Southeast Asian anti-aging cream. Consumers and human placenta encapsulation providers cite medical properties and spirituality as reasons for eating and encapsulating the placenta: the ability to connect spiritually with the baby, reduce postpartum depression, and restore iron and other nutrient levels after childbirth. The placenta gains other cultural and commodity meanings when companies such as Japan Bio Products use placentas in their cosmetic lines, citing the placenta's unique ability to repair damaged and ailing skin with whitening benefits, in order to ensure a perfect, bright complexion. In the case study, I illustrate how placenta bioproducts draw upon nationalized imaginaries when, for instance, Japanese human placentas are framed as good quality products and marketed as 100 percent Japanese placenta extract.[8] Meanwhile the Danish organic pigs' placentas that turn into an ingredient in the anti-aging cream produced by the Japanese company Hirosophy are positioned as being healthier than humans living in urban environments.[9] The chapter is based on marketing material, interviews with women who consume their placenta, interviews with Danish midwives who regularly handle the placenta, visits to a major Japanese placenta pharmaceutical and cosmetics company, and an interview with the company BHJ located in Southern Denmark, which picks up, handles, and distributes pig placentas to the Asian pharmaceutical market.

The three case studies jointly show how reproductive donations move out of the realm of reproductive waste and into that of reproductive value in different ways. In my conclusion, I discuss the cultural politics and the moral limits associated with the ways that global fluids move in and out of the marketplace. As noted by Radin (1996), reproductive donations are contested commodities. They do not begin as commodities but enter in and out of different commodity states, as Parry (2007) similarly argues. Tissue extraction and biotechnical processing and techniques enable biological matter to become valuable in new ways, or, as noted by Waldby and

Mitchell, "Waste material which may appear as the very opposite of value in one context can become the starting point for the generation of significant degrees of value in another" (Waldby and Mitchell 2006: 84). The three cases presented in *Global Fluids* illustrate how biovalue is accumulated in different ways while prioritizing different geopolitical contexts as well (Japan, Spain, Denmark, and the Netherlands). They show how reproductive matter moves from individual providers through reproductive technologies, clinical expertise, and industrial processes, in each entanglement gaining cultural value focusing on the performances that go into these forms of biocommerce and positioning reproductive donations as nature reinvented.

In the conclusion, I turn to the development of feminist cultural politics of reproductive donations and raise the following questions: What things may or may not be (commercially) exchanged? And why do some reproductive donations lead troubled lives while others swiftly enter a globalized resource economy? Feminist scholars have aptly criticized what they position as the market in reproduction (human eggs, sperm, and wombs), fragmenting women into sellable reproductive parts (Dickenson 2009; Scheper-Hughes 2015). In fact, providing the pharmaceutical industry with one's urine or placenta may at first glance appear less market-like. To engage this discussion, I turn to feminist perspectives on commodification, and I challenge what I see as the false (and unproductive) dichotomy between the gift and market economies. Instead, I argue that oocytes, urine, and placenta move in and out of different commodity states, and I note that feminist cultural politics on reproductive waste and value will benefit from looking beyond *what* is exchanged to *the acts* through which certain parts become exchangeable and enter different commodity states (Malmqvist 2012; Hoeyer 2013). Consequently, the feminist cultural analyst must respond to the following questions: What practices are involved when particular reproductive parts are exchanged? And what are the intended as well as unintended effects of these practices? Rose extends this argument when he stresses that reproductive markets not only create new possibilities for wealth but embody, generate, and perhaps even reconfigure ethical values (Rose 2007: 152).

Through engagement with feminist scholarship and drawing upon an assemblage of different empirical material, *Global Fluids* seeks to develop a distinct feminist cultural analytical contribution that addresses not only the economics of reproductive donations but also the ways that reproductive donations engage the hopes and dreams of providers, businesses, technologies, consumers, and recipients; I therefore center the ways that reproductive donations are always already entangled and embedded in social and cultural relations. So the goal of this book is not to separate reproductive donations from biology but to illustrate how reproductive donations are jointly constituted and fabricated in the entanglements between nature and culture, nature and commerce, and nature and science, contributing to the ongoing feminist debates on the cultural politics of reproduction.

Notes

1. The sharing of breast milk as a form of donation is, for instance, seen on the "Only the Breast: A Community for Moms" website available at: http://www.onlythebreast.com (retrieved January 2016).
2. While the scientific evidence seems to vary, some reports do emphasize the ability for Pregnyl to be used for purposes other than ovarian stimulation. For example, see Zehr (2017) for a description of the use of Pregnyl in weight loss programs.
3. Japan Bio Products international affiliations can be seen on the company's online profile: Japan Bio Products Co., Ltd., "Company Profile," http://jbpglobal.placenta.co.jp/about/company/ (retrieved January 2016).
4. Professor Ayo Wahlberg, University of Copenhagen, introduced me to the concept of assemblage ethnography and contributed to my thinking on this topic. In his forthcoming (2018) book, Wahlberg uses the term assemblage ethnography as a ways of describing relations—whether regional or global—that appear in a particular site.
5. An exception to this is Wahlberg's forthcoming (2018) book.
6. Reference is here made to the Explanatory Report on the European Treaty Series—No. 164, retrieved September 2017 from https://rm.coe.int/16800ccde5.
7. In the first Danish law on assisted reproduction, transporting oocytes out of the country is deemed illegal. The text reads: "It is not permitted to bring unfertilized or fertilized human oocytes that in this country have been extracted, for the purposes of artificial insemination or research, abroad" (retrieved September 2017 from https://www.retsinformation.dk/Forms/R0710.aspx?id=84963 § 16). This part of the law was changed in 2012 largely due to a Danish couple who had fertilized oocytes stored in Denmark yet were living abroad. Consequently, the 2012 law on assisted reproduction does not contain this limitation: https://www.retsinformation.dk/Forms/R0710.aspx?id=141094 (retrieved September 2017).

8. An example of this type of product is Miccosmo's "White Label: Premium Placenta Essence," http://www.miccosmo.co.jp/english/wl.html (retrieved January 2016).
9. This can, for instance, be seen in Hirosophy's presentation of their use of Danish placentas available on their website: http://www.hirosophy.co.jp/ (retrieved January 2016).

Chapter 1

Scholarly Conversation

The Danish pig farmer bags and recycles fresh and warm placentas from Danish pigs before rushing them off to the refrigerator. This chapter theorizes how reproductive donations are removed from individual bodies as waste material and turn into (new) valuable bioproducts. To begin, however, I outline a more general feminist cultural analytical perspective on the ways that rhetoric, affects, and material "things" entangle to produce particular understandings of the reproductive body. Following this presentation, I turn to the ways that reproductive donations—in this case, oocytes, placentas, and urine—are removed from individual female bodies and, through clinical or industrial practices, engage the hopes and dreams of the predominantly female consumers. As will become clear, mobility does not only pertain to the ways in which reproductive donations move physically. Rather, mobility refers to the ways in which reproduction enters into new value relations as affective bioproducts, engaging, for example, with dreams of future children or the desire for youthful-looking skin or healthy, energetic maternal bodies.

In this chapter I use what has become known as the *mobility turn* to position my own work (Sheller and Urry 2004), and I outline the scholarship of feminist theorists to discuss how reproductive donations are globalized and gain regenerative and consumer value (Franklin et al. 2000; Lash and Lury 2007; Waldby and Cooper 2008; Waldby 2006a, 2006b). I am interested in theorizing the ways that reproductive donations (oocytes, placentas, and urine) move, as well as how people (patients, providers, clinical experts) and various technologies (clinical webpages, social networking sites, containers, transportation, freezers, extraction techniques, visualization technologies) facilitate mobility. I argue that reproductive donations are entangled in scientific developments and the geopolitics of the fertility industry. To this extent, mobility is by no means value-neutral. Quite to the contrary, cultural values are embedded in the ways in which reproductive donations, people, and technologies move. Reproductive mobility, then, frequently works together with the neoliberal restructuring of global economies (Vora 2015: 6). To understand this complexity, I first outline feminist cultural analysis as a pertinent analytical perspective employed throughout this book, and I then turn to a more in-depth theorizing of reproductive waste and value prior to presenting my approach to reproductive mobility and reproduction as global/local practices.

Feminist Cultural Analysis of Reproduction

Feminist cultural analysis of reproduction constitutes a productive framework for understanding how reproduction is inscribed with cultural values throughout the processes of visualization, marketing, extraction, industrialization, commodification, and consumption. But what does a feminist cultural analytical perspective look like? How does it differ from other analytical methods used by feminist historians, sociologists, anthropologists, medical scientists, or ethicists? In this section I take a closer look at feminist cultural analysis centering rhetoric, affects, and material "things," and I explain the workings of feminist cultural analysis through brief examinations of three Danish campaigns. In this first subsection on rhetorical and communication analysis tools, I include the Copenhagen fertility campaign Have You Counted Your Eggs Today? (2015), and in the section on affects and materiality, I turn to the campaigns of the Danish travel agent, Spies: Do It for Denmark and Do It for Mom (2013 and 2015). Feminist cultural analysis situates gender as an analytical enabling device and, as will become evident in chapters 2–4, this analytical perspective will grant me strategies through which various configurations of reproductive waste and value can be understood.

Feminist Rhetorical and Communication Analysis

Have you counted your eggs today? In 2015, the city of Copenhagen together with one of the leading public fertility clinics in Denmark launched a major campaign aimed at encouraging women (and men) to have children in their twenties. With a headline written in pink, a white background, and pinkish-looking chicken eggs, the campaign informed women that "your chance of becoming a mother is twice as high at the age of 25 compared to 35." In contrast, the campaign directed at Copenhagen men featured a blue background, a large group of normal-looking, light-blue-colored sperm (moving in the same direction), a headline ("Are they swimming too slow?"), and the informational blurb "40% have reduced sperm quality. It can take time to become a father." Throughout this subsection I rely on the Copenhagen campaign to illustrate the workings of feminist rhetorical and communication analysis, and I pay particular attention to the production of three rhetorical configurations that will reappear as analytical constructs in the chapters to come: the neoliberal, the entrepreneurial, and the philanthropic body.

To feminist rhetorical scholars (Lay et al. 2000; Martin 1991), rhetorical practices construct the reproductive body and its parts. Rhetorical scholars note that reproduction is constructed in and through communication (Foss et al. 1999, 2004). Feminist rhetorical analysis includes an examination of word choices, arguments, warrants, claims, visuals, and mediated forms of communication to examine how they gain persuasiveness at various sites. With regard to the Copenhagen campaign, the strategic use of the word "you" in the "Have **you** counted your eggs today?" effectively places reproductive responsibility on the shoulders of individual young women. The directness with which women are hailed toward an egg count did not go unnoticed, however. Following the campaign, young Copenhagen women responded in social media with photos of chicken eggs and what may be framed as "Get the city out of our ovaries" rhetoric. For example, one woman commenting upon her choice to upload a photo of four chicken eggs writes, "Dear city of Copenhagen. I have four eggs left and 8 months till I graduate. Is there anything else you want to interfere in?" (Mølgaard 2015). As these examples demonstrate, meanings are rhetorically produced and negotiated in particular communication contexts (Lay et al. 2000).

By viewing reproduction in the light of its rhetorical features, a feminist cultural analyst privileges an understanding of reproduction as constituted in and through communication. The rhetorical analyst pays attention to how key rhetorical terms involve both high-frequency terms (terms that are frequently used) and high-intensity terms (terms that have significant affective value) (Foss 1984). According to Foss (1984), this analytical method is particularly adept in granting insights into what goes on, including the gendered practices that are enacted in and through communication.

To return to the Copenhagen campaign, while the female reproductive body rhetorically gets constructed as a neoliberal, individually responsible body (who has to count, protect, and manage her eggs), the vocabulary used in the "Are they swimming too slow?" campaign constructs infertility as less within the control of the individual male and more as a point of general awareness ("It can take time to become a father"). Thus, while reproductive aging is demonized in the campaign directed toward women (twenty-five years of age is twice as good as thirty-five), neither age nor health appears to be of concern to the men, although optimal sperm is understood as fast swimmers. The campaign is rhetorically about speed and mobility, while visually, because it collectively shows a large group of healthy-looking sperm cells, it cements the idea that male fertility is about quantity (and endless amounts of sperm cells) and good-looking swimmers.

To feminist rhetorical and communication scholars, rhetoric involves a fixing of meaning, a reiteration of conventions, and a materializing of performativity (Kroløkke 2012; Pollock 1999). Pollock (1999) illustrates this in her research on women's birth stories. She notes how birth stories can be understood as risky performances and situated as "carefully-guarded doubles" that reveal and manage dichotomies, such as those between nature/culture, life/death, public/private, pleasure/pain (Pollock 1999: 248). Pollock (1999) argues that in their birth stories, women reveal the meaning of birth, including conventional norms and expectations. Rhetorical and communication analyses help deconstruct scientific storytelling in order to note how language represents the body, while also revealing how rhetorical frames influence cultural and gendered attitudes on reproduction. For example, Nadesan and Trethewey (2000) echo this when they show how gendered strategies of success are frequently understood within the rhetorical frame of the enterprising subject. Meanwhile, Markens (2007) notes how reproduction within the context of gestational surrogacy gets positioned in one of two tropes: the "plight of the infertile couples" or the "baby-selling" frames, producing very different understandings of the altruistic surrogate body or the commoditized body and simultaneously promoting very different calls for social intervention.

Key to feminist rhetorical analysis is being attentive to the ways that metaphors provide leaps between different conceptual domains (Lakoff and Johnson 1980; Jacobsen 2004). Martin (1987) eloquently illustrates how cultural assumptions are embedded in scientific understandings of the female reproductive body as a "small business," as a "factory," as an "information-transmission system," or as a "machine." The metaphor of the body as a small business prioritizes the ways that the reproductive body balances itself (through in- and outflows) yet tends, according to Martin (1987), to position medical doctors as managers and supervisors delegating the worker position to women. This is similarly the case when viewing the body as a factory or a machine in which women are laborers, guided and managed by (male) doctors, and children are products of reproduction (Martin 1987). Again, in the case of the Copenhagen campaign, the metaphor of the slow swimmers reinforces the notion of the desirable male reproductive body as a competitive one (fast and strong). Characteristic of this rhetoric is the overall tendency to stress the ability to reproduce as a normative and even valuable act, and so failing to reproduce, whether due to infertility, menstruation, no swimmers, crabby eggs, aging, or simply out of a desire to remain child-free, is understood as "production gone awry, making products of no use, not to specification, unsalable, wasted, scrap" (Martin 1987: 46).

The attention to rhetoric reveals other metaphors as well. To Franklin et al. (2000), the metaphor of the body as an ecosystem replaces the more simplistic notion of the body as a machine. When positioned in a neoliberal context, however, the body as an ecosystem must simultaneously be seen to involve the individualized responsibility of "keeping oneself informed, [and] the duty to calculate risk" (Franklin et al. 2000: 41). This is readily seen in the Copenhagen campaign as well, when young female bodies are purposefully disciplined and oriented toward a particular temporality of reproduction: have your children early. As also noted by Nadesan and Trethewey, the move toward what I position as an entrepreneurial body is an egalitarian ideal in which the individual is responsible for managing her own reproductive success, including, in the case of the Copenhagen campaign, counting and thereby exercising the responsible management of one's fertility, which now completely resides in the eggs. This is most notably reiterated in the case of egg freezing, when women take up an entrepreneurial position by freezing a batch of their eggs and so engage in a form of "responsible" reproductive citizenship (Carroll and Kroløkke 2017).

Consequently, from a rhetorical point of view, reproductive fluids or organs do not have innate biological meanings. Rather, their meanings are acquired in social interactions and through communication practices. As already witnessed, this is swiftly illustrated in the existing feminist and cultural analytical scholarship on the reproductive body (Martin 1991, 1987). For Martin (1987), medical metaphors on the reproductive body reveal how constructions of the body and its parts are gendered and located in specific cultural contexts. Menstruation, for example, gets positioned as unclean matter expelled from the body, while menopause is framed rhetorically as a product of "unresponsive" or "senile" ovaries (Martin 1987: 42). Martin (1987) argues that rhetorical (and cultural) emphasis on production within reproduction explains why oocytes in the dominant narrative take on a more passive role compared to sperm, as well as why the menopausal body becomes less valuable as its reproductive power ceases to exist. As argued by Martin, "Far from being *produced* like sperm is, they (ovarian follicles) seem to merely sit on the shelf, as it were, slowly degenerating and aging like overstocked inventory" (Martin 1987: 49). The Copenhagen campaign aptly speaks of this. Here six chicken eggs are completely or at least partially shown. They appear static, fragile, situated side by side. In contrast, the potentially "poor" swimmers display activity: they all look healthy and swim collectively. While the message indicates a concern for "slow" swimmers, the rhetoric that it takes time to become a father and the sheer numbers of sperm contrast with the more fear-driven rhetoric in the campaign directed toward women in whom there seems to be a very limited number of eggs present. Thus, while men are made aware that a large number of adult men have poor sperm quality, women's fertility seemingly resides in their eggs, and as women age, their fertility is running out literally as well as figuratively.

Attention to rhetoric provides the analyst with tools for understanding how reproduction is rhetorically granted value. It illustrates how particular reproductive paths and reproductive bodies are made to appear legitimate, even natural, and it suggests that words and rhetorical tropes activate certain realities, and as such they are never arbitrary but, rather, indicative of various cultural shifts. As noted by Jacobsen, "Tropes are closely interwoven within the basic structures and grids of power in a society" (Jacobsen 2004: 60). While I have emphasized the rhetorical construction of the neoliberal and entrepreneurial reproductive body, in chapters 2–4 another rhetorical construct appears; namely, that of the philanthropic body where the reproductive body's regenerative value is positioned within a gifting resource economy. The philanthropic body maximizes itself not only as necessary to achieve personal benefits but also to enact social commitments embedded in giving someone else the chance of motherhood. The rhetorical constructions of the neoliberal, the entrepreneurial, and the philanthropic body construct an understanding of the female body as having choice and agency. In this manner, rhetorical constructs on the body (and its parts) compete to achieve dominance, while they also draw upon gendered, racial, sexualized, and national understandings of reproduction, including the idea that reproducing one's genes is the very essence of life.

As demonstrated in this first subsection, reproduction is contested and negotiated rhetorically. Having briefly explained how rhetoric and communication play an integral role in the formulation of feminist cultural analysis, I turn now to a discussion of analytical strategies that examines what affects and matter do, and I use the Danish Spies travel campaigns Do It for Denmark and Do It for Mom to help illustrate the analytical insights gained from affects and materiality.

Feminist Affect and Materialist Analyses

Sitting alone on a bench in the park, an older Danish white woman with short, white hair, glasses, and sensible clothes looks longingly at another similarly aged woman who stands next to what appears to be her young granddaughter. Unlike the woman alone on the bench, this older woman smiles as the young child throws bread crumbs to a small group of ducks. The Danish travel campaign Do It for Mom is a call for Danish could-be grandmothers to take action and send their children on an "active" (read: fertile) vacation. If they (the adult children) won't do it for their country, the video claims, surely they will do it for mom. Do It for Mom is the Danish travel company Spies's creative effort at mixing reproduction with travel. The company earlier produced a Do It for Denmark commercial in which Emma, a tall, slender, white, Danish woman with long blonde hair, is in Paris together with her unnamed boyfriend. Emma was in fact conceived, we hear, in Paris, and the travel company notes that Danes have 46 percent more sex when on vacation, thus making a romantic city holiday the ideal solution to what is framed as the growing Danish fertility problem. Both videos mix what is naturalized as societal calls for more (white) Danish children, statistical evidence documenting the falling birth rates, clinical evidence that the release of endorphins leads to an increased desire for sex with mostly young, attractive, able-bodied, and—in the case of the Do It for Mom video—sweaty, wet, white, heterosexual, lusting partners. Each video ends with an acknowledgment that not everyone can match this ideal. Do It for Denmark includes an older couple (they have already "done their duty," we hear) and a gay couple (positioned as not being able to perform "the duty"), while Do It for Mom includes a young, white man who still lives at home with his mom. In this subsection I turn to the workings of feminist affective and material perspectives, and I include brief analyses noting how affects of love and desire in these videos, along with technology, sweat, and wetness, serve to construct and naturalize very particular understandings of reproductive bodies.

Focusing on "the emotionality of texts" (Ahmed 2004: 12), Ahmed's poststructuralist approach to affects is at first glance closely aligned with rhetoric and communication theory, yet it extends beyond the realm of rhetoric to the ways that "emotions move between bodies" (Ahmed 2004: 117). To Ahmed, affects or emotions circulate to create particular effects such as naturalizing certain bodies as rightful reproductive citizens. Frequently displayed in metaphors and figures of speech, Ahmed argues that emotions are performative, meaning that emotions produce particular understandings of reality, or, as she contends, "Emotions *do things,* and they align individuals with communities through the very intensity of their attachments" (Ahmed 2004: 119). In Do It for Mom, the male voiceover makes the falling birth rates personal in that they affect grandmothers the most ("But those that suffer the most are perhaps the mothers who will never experience having a grandchild"), which combined with the fact that this older woman is physically alone, inactive, has a worried look, and longingly directs her visual gaze to a young, white child, naturalizes the desire for a particular grandchild. In fact, the urge to become a grandmother gets positioned in the video as being "grandma-broody." Affects are, as noted by Ahmed, neither within nor outside the individual; rather, affects gain their performative effect through the ways that they circulate. In the video, the desire for a grandchild (here conceptualized as an object of happiness), coupled with loneliness, works to make the making of babies while on vacation appear necessary, even natural.

Characteristic of this analytical interest in affects is a tendency to view emotions as rhetorical, as well as material, embodied resources. To Sheller and Urry, the physical body can be viewed as an affective vehicle "through which we sense place and movement, and construct emotional choreographies" (Sheller and Urry 2006: 216). As argued by Hochschild (1979), emotional labor is governed by social rules and is stratified by race, sex, age, and class. It involves making emotions match feeling rules that "are not completely of their own making" (Hochschild 1979: 563). Within the context of the transnational fertility clinic, the growing number of fertility coordinators constitutes an interesting case in point. Frequently young women with no prior reproductive or medical education, fertility coordinators arrive at the clinic (some of them from the tourism industry) not only to coordinate travel and treatment but also to emotionally manage the intended parents' hopes, fears, and dreams of having a baby. In this manner, affects circulate to produce particular effects. In the case of the international coordinators, they re-naturalize intended parents' longing for a child as innate and biological. Similarly, the Spanish clinical marketing material and doctors position egg providers as innately friendly and gift-giving young women (Kroløkke 2014). The Do It for Mom and Do It for Denmark campaigns similarly naturalize reproduction within an affective economy, in which reproduction is both innate and a form of good citizenship. In Do It for Mom, the could-be grandmother's previous maternal work testifies to her inherent maternal qualities, which serve to support her legitimatized desire for a genetic-related grandchild. In contrast, in the Do It for Denmark video, affective labor is made to appear a patriotic ideal, in which love and care for the nation work to make the (re)production of ethnic (white) Danish children appear natural and desirable.

The analytical interest in affects extends beyond the rhetorical realm into the sensory and sensuous realms, as well as the ways that bodies physically move. As noted by Waskul and Vannini (2008), sense-making is a type of somatic work, and, similarly, (in)activity causes particular understandings of the reproductive body. In Do It for Denmark, we watch Emma as she visits the hotel room where she was conceived. In response to the male voice-over comment "if only these walls could talk," she pulls up her nose as if smelling her parents' sexual activities. In Do It for Mom, activity comes to signify respectable and deserving reproductive bodies. The video informs the viewers that activity releases endorphins and creates more sex drive, yet this material flow is restricted to the mostly or at least partially undressed young, middle-class, attractive couple. Whereas the could-be grandmother is inactive, her memories of helping to teach her son to walk or ride a bicycle are characteristically active and are portrayed in the video as "happy moments." Today, her activity seemingly includes pressing the button to make a contribution toward her son's vacation and jumping for joy, together with other hopeful grandmothers, as the imagined flight takes off to its fertile destination.

Feminist scholars of science studies and, in particular, material-semiotic understandings of the body destabilize positivist notions of science (Barad 2003; Haraway 1991). In bringing a materialist perspective to feminist cultural analyses, the researcher extends her inquiries to technological apparatuses, sensory and material practices (Åsberg and Lykke 2010). Technological developments are seen as pivotal to individual experiences and practices. As noted by Thompson (2005), the ontological interrelationship between the individual and the environment has profound implications on how individuals narrate their experiences. Berglund and Lundin (2012) have similarly elaborated on this point by demonstrating the desire of Swedish kidney patients to disrupt their dependency on dialysis machines in order to travel abroad for kidney donations. Understanding how reproduction moves and becomes involved with different cultural understandings, scientific processes, technological developments, and physical equipment (e.g., containers, petri dishes, freezers, and machines) shapes how reproduction comes to matter and gets to be understood (Adrian 2010; Thompson 2005). In Do It for Mom and Do It for Denmark, reproductive technologies are strikingly absent—and this in spite of the fact that one out of twelve Danish children today are estimated to have been born with the assistance of IVF. Instead, reproduction is re-situated as exclusively "natural" involving heteronormative, attractive, young, white, middle-class bodies. An exception to this is the online ovulation test, which, in the Do It for Denmark video, promises to assist the interested couples in determining not only when to have sex but when to travel. Other technologies and material practices include an empty playground (which reminds us of the need for more children), different attractive and exotic settings (a holiday in the sun, a pool, a gym, Paris), recognizable sights that get imbued with sexual overtones (the Eiffel Tower and Moulin Rouge), as well as wetness (wet bodies coming out of the pool in slow motion) and sweat (bodies working out and bodies having sex). Attention to the material and sensory/sensuous environment so readily available in the videos illustrates how reproduction, when it involves particular (young, attractive, white, heterosexual) bodies, is resituated as innate and natural.

Attention to materiality necessitates a move to the ways that practices are enacted (Mol 2002). In her groundbreaking book *The Body Multiple: Ontology in Medical Practice,* Mol calls for a practice-oriented approach that "stubbornly takes notice of the techniques that make things visible, audible, tangible, knowable. She may talk bodies—but she never forgets about microscopes" (Mol 2002: 33). To Mol (2002), practices are enacted, meaning that objects are never singular nor exclusively subjects or objects; rather, they are created in very specific acts. While feminist scholars within rhetorical and affect-analytical approaches tend to use the performance and performativity concepts in discussing what affects and rhetoric *do*, Mol (2002) deliberately distances herself from the performance metaphor and prefers the verb "enact" that assists her, she argues, in deconstructing the object/subject dichotomy. As she notes, "This suggests that activities take place—but leaves the actors vague. It also suggests that in the act, and only then and there, something is—being enacted" (Mol 2002: 33). This relationship between the material and the discursive is reiterated in the scholarship of Barad as one of mutual entailment, and includes viewing rhetoric, affects, and material "things":

> Neither is articulated/articulable in the absence of the other; matter and meaning are mutually articulated. Neither discursive practices nor material phenomena are ontologically or epistemologically prior. Neither can be explained in terms of the other. Neither has privileged status in determining the other. (Barad 2003: 822)

Attention to the ways that affects, materiality (such as technologies, places, visualization techniques, and instruments), mobility, and senses come together in particular acts provides the analyst with insights into how reproductive bodies are constituted and, at times, naturalized. In Do It for Mom, the respectable reproductive body is a young, physically fit, white, heterosexual body, while in Do It for Denmark, it is entangled with pride and love for not just any nation but, in the case of this campaign, the Danish welfare state. In both campaigns, the desire to genetically reproduce is re-naturalized through the visual engagement with popularized images of sperm cells and a large, glowing egg cell (which has an uncanny resemblance to the sun). When these affects and material "things" are situated together with scientific visual representations of the release of endorphins, the sun, sweat, wet bodies, lust, and love, it comes together to make the act of heterosexual reproduction seem desirable and innate. I turn now to suggest how this feminist cultural analytical perspective can inform our understanding of reproductive donations.

Feminist Cultural Analysis on Reproductive Donations

In formulating a wide-angled analytical perspective, I stress how feminist cultural analysis examines and documents the ways that reproductive donations move, including their various entanglements with technologies, ideas, emotions, images, words, and metaphors, as well as how they may become idioms across different domains and in different assemblages. In what follows, I briefly discuss a feminist cultural analytical perspective on reproductive donations.

An emphasis on affects and matter, as well as rhetoric and communication, is necessary for an appropriate understanding of the ways that reproductive donations turn into bioproducts through various paths of circulation and commodification, while they simultaneously take on gendered, racial, national, sexual, and class stratifications and deploy and transfigure various understandings of what comes to constitute nature. As is clear from this presentation, reproductive donations are not merely rhetorical, discursive, or affective. They are physical matter as well. A placenta may be rhetorically framed as "biohazardous material," or as "a nutritional supplement," yet it is also fleshy, bloody, and stringy matter. Placentas exit the body and are shown, photographed, held, carried, and scrutinized. Similarly, oocytes are reproductive matter. Egg cells can be extracted and visualized, and urine (avoided by most, yet fetishized by some) can be seen, smelled, and felt. Oocytes are extracted from the body, while placentas and urine are expelled from the body, at times with medical evidence documenting hormone levels and signs of pregnancy, an unhealthy lifestyle, or illness. At the same time, placenta consumption and even oocyte donation draw upon and reiterate existing kin relations. In the case of placenta consumption, an affectionate mother–child bond is key to the desire to perform this form of responsible (intensive) motherhood. Similarly, in cases of oocyte donation, a biological (if not genetic) bond is stressed when oocyte recipients articulate the importance of their own reproductive desires and biological experiences (e.g., pregnancy, birth, and nursing). Moreover, in these narratives, oocyte recipients and birthing mothers are the rightful biological, if not genetic, parents of children (Kroløkke 2012, 2014). A turn to materiality empirically necessitates a turn to places, technologies, equipment, modes of transportation (vans, cars, and planes), and new communication technologies, for example.

Combining this interest in rhetoric, communication, affects, and materiality has profound implications for doing research. It centers other questions and curiosities, raising questions such as: Why do Spanish laboratories operate in dimmed lighting during in vitro fertilization procedures when Danish laboratories are fully lit? Why do Spanish clinics insist that oocyte recipients walk through a floor mat full of glue to remove all outside matter before treatment, when Danish fertility clinics have no such concern? Why does sperm donation, in a London-based clinic, take place in the basement of the fertility clinic, when the center of the clinic is on the ground floor? In short, how do such material practices, locations, and technologies entangle with reproductive donations to produce particular understandings and lived realities? In the case of placentas, Japan Bio Products, a Japanese company producing medical and cosmetic products made from placenta, retrieves more than four thousand human placentas a month in company vans and transforms them into medical injections and anti-aging and whitening lotions. In a different process, oocytes are retrieved from provider bodies, placed in petri dishes, frozen, fertilized, labeled with the female recipient's name, and later brought back to life through new visualization technologies that display the developing embryo on an embryonic film (van de Wiel 2016). Through such practices, gametes, urine, and placentas cease to belong to the provider bodies from which they came and circulate into the transnational fertility industry.

In turning to affects of love, care, and desire, the analyst might note how reproductive donations get invested in particular affective strategies. In the case of transnational oocyte donation, female oocyte recipients are invested in framing oocyte providing as an altruistic act, as this works to erase any potential discomfort associated with exchanging oocytes for compensation (Kroløkke 2014). Similarly, affects of desperation combined with fear, due to years of waiting for a kidney transplant in Sweden, produce a particular directionality in the transnational traveling of Swedish first-generation immigrants (born outside of Sweden) and kidney recipients who choose to travel abroad for transplantation (Berglund and Lundin 2012). Moreover, affects such as love and disgust constitute another understanding of reproductive donations. This is evident in the case of the placenta: When placenta consumption is framed as a loving act and a form of good mothering (an affectionate, caring, maternal choice), the placenta gets positioned as more akin to a heart than a liver. In sharp contrast, an affect such as disgust situates placenta consumption as less of a spiritual experience than a cannibalistic one, resituating the placenta as first and foremost meaty, bloody, organic matter. A focus on affects helps to illustrate how love, care, desire, and disgust produce and re-naturalize very different understandings of reproductive donations.

Having highlighted how rhetoric, communication, affects, and materiality constitute vital components of the feminist cultural analytical perspective employed throughout this book, I turn now to theories that discuss how reproductive donations move from being classified as reproductive waste to being understood as reproductive value.

On Reproductive Waste and Value

> Waste material, which may appear as the very opposite of value in one context, can be the starting point for the generation of significant degrees of value in another. Hence, one of the fundamental movements of any successful form of economy is the circulation of waste objects from unprofitable to profitable contexts, where they can be resignified and redeployed. (Waldby and Mitchell 2006: 84)

Waste and value are dynamic and contested categories (Strasser 1999; Hawkins 2003; Douglas [1966] 1984; Waldby and Mitchell 2006; Moser 2002). In the case of reproductive donations, human oocytes are embedded with varying and shifting meanings, as they cross not only time and space but also varying cultural terrains (Bharadwaj 2008; Thompson 2005). They are "bio-objectified" (Holmberg et al. 2011) as "necessary genetic material," "surplus matter," "spare parts," and even as the promise or potential of intelligent, beautiful future babies (Kroløkke 2014). Bio-objectification involves not only economic exchanges but also a moral economy in which "things" are deemed commodities at certain times but not at others (Kopytoff 1986). I return to this issue in the conclusion, but for now I note that despite historical evidence to the contrary (slaves, sex workers, or organ trafficking, for example), humans, embryos, and organs have frequently been framed as what should not be commoditized. This has been especially true as far as reproductive tissue and organs are concerned. Kopytoff puts this succinctly when he states that "the realm of human reproduction is one in which the difference between persons and things is particularly difficult to define, defying all attempts at drawing a simple line where there is a natural continuum" (Kopytoff 1986: 86). In this section, I discuss the processes involved in waste and value formations, and along with Waldby and Mitchell (2006) I argue that, in fact, it is the very ability to be labeled as "waste" that enables reproductive donations to gain new value and enter into new domains.

But how do we come to understand bodily waste? Waldby and Mitchell pose that ideas on waste are integral in understanding the ways that tissue in one assemblage comes to be deemed "waste"—insignificant to the person it comes from—and is subsequently recycled within "the infrastructures of capitalism and commodity culture" (Waldby and Mitchell 2006: 83). Understanding human bodily waste in light of its ontological significance is necessary to conceptualize the ways that human tissue becomes exchangeable. Examples include urine, sweat, and skin particles that are expelled from the body and, upon being expelled, have little significance to the body that they came from (Waldby and Mitchell 2006). More troubled exchanges include tissue or parts that are surgically removed, such as aborted fetuses, tumors, oocytes, or infant foreskins, that similarly enter into scientific or commercial exchanges (Waldby and Mitchell 2006). To Moster (2002), waste takes on a technical, an economic, a historical and an aesthetic discourse. Waste can be understood as "decay" (that which has passively fallen off), as "rejection" (that which has been actively detached), as "death" (that which no longer exists), as "negativity" (that which is disgusting), or as zero-value (that which is outside the realm of economic and cultural value) (Moster 2002: 87; Hawkins 2003). This is in contrast to tissue or parts that have been deemed integral and necessary to the body, such as organs, skin, or limbs (Waldby and Mitchell 2006).

Bodily waste is not value neutral. Some tissue and bodily parts conjure up feelings of disgust or repulsion (Waldby and Mitchell 2006). This is notably the case with human feces that, as Hawkins (2003) illustrates it, disrupt the "boundaries between the body and its others, public and private, truth and concealment, state and environment, and, of course, pure and impure" (Hawkins 2003: 42). Developing a politics of disturbance, Hawkins employs Foucault's understanding of biopower to the technologies of waste, arguing how, in the case of shit, the "category of the unacceptable demands extensive description of how to exclude it" (Hawkins 2003: 44). Shit is managed by positioning it away from the public and within the private realm of the household. Unclean transactions have become privatized, or as noted by Hawkins, "Money and shit are distanced from the state, both standing for the private realm and both enhancing the state's aura of public goodness and benevolence" (Hawkins 2003: 44). When shit is repositioned to unfold in the private realm, it is out of public sight and smell.

From an anthropological and sociological perspective, waste is understood as matter out of place (Douglas [1966] 1984; Strasser 1999). To Susan Strasser (1999), waste is created through sorting, and it has a spatial dimension as well, when it gets physically moved outside, positioned out of view. In Douglas's ([1966] 1984) early and groundbreaking research, dirt is not innately wasteful material but, rather, out-of-place matter. Douglas states that the quest to create order is evidence of a very specific desire to create value out of disorder: "In chasing dirt, in papering, decorating, tidying, we are not governed by anxiety to escape disease, but are positively reordering our environment, making it conform to an idea" (Douglas [1966] 1984: 3). According to Douglas ([1966] 1984), the search for purity is productive for understanding waste in general, as well as what the body expels as reproductive waste in particular (e.g., urine, menstrual blood, and placentas). In her perspective, the ordering involved becomes "an attempt to force experience into logical categories of non-contradiction" (Douglas [1966] 1984: 200). Reproductive donations swiftly illustrate this as well. In the case of the placenta, for example, when exiting the body, it becomes matter in need of a (new) place. Putting the placenta in the hospital bin or in the freezer creates a particular understanding of it as trash material, while circulating it into the larger bioeconomy enables other transactions to take place, in which placentas become a food commodity, hormone extract, placenta money, or anti-aging product, for example.

Reproductive waste gets new economic and cultural value through a process of recycling. Waldby and Mitchell (2006) persuasively illustrate how the tissue economy is contingent upon the circulation of "waste" tissue into scientific and commercial undertakings. Similarly, in their introduction to what is understood as the cultural economy of waste, Hawkins and Muecke stress that waste is unable to escape the "value-laden circuits of production and consumption" (Hawkins and Muecke 2003: ix). The North American campaign Recycle Yourself serves as a case in point.[1] In the quest for more organ donors, the campaign promotes "recycling life" through compelling recipient stories, such as eight-year-old Lindsay who, upon receiving a heart, has also been given a "second chance."[2] Whereas donors are united and made to appear anonymous under the rubric of "recycling life," recipients are visually portrayed, as well as textually documented in individual, personalized recipient stories.

Waste and value are dynamic processes. Throughout this book, reproductive donations are not intrinsically waste or intrinsically of value. In fact, reproductive donations become waste and value when they enter into particular assemblages and move through various institutional structures, such as from the individual woman to the institutional structure of a hospital or clinic, a research institution, laboratory, or a corporate entity (Frow 2003). As noted by Hawkins and Muecke, the interest and ability to recycle waste illustrates how waste and value are "neither the province of the economy nor of culture, but are constantly transacted between the two in multiple sites and regimes" (Hawkins and Muecke 2003: xi). Similarly,

Waldby and Mitchell argue that recycling is an economic move and involves "relocating waste to other regimes of value where it does productive work" (Waldby and Mitchell 2006: 84). In fact, this move from waste to value is exactly the reason why Waldby and Mitchell position human biological tissue as neither a gift nor exclusively a commodity; rather, waste establishes a third category and "mediates and informs" the understanding of gifts and commodities in complex ways (Waldby and Mitchell 2006: 85). I will return to this discussion in my conclusion.

What has the appearance of waste may intersect with what Rajan (2017) calls biological capital in several ways. Rajan (2017) uses the concept of biocapital in his analyses of the U.S. biotech industry and the Indian state. According to him, genetic material gets translated into an information science and therefore, invariably, gets entangled with promissory capital and value. While he views biocapital as a "technoscientific enterprise" (Rajan 2017: 111) in centering the "grammar of biocapital" (Rajan 2017: 110), he privileges how the rhetoric of biocapital is frequently entangled with a future-oriented value. As he notes, "To generate value in the present to make a certain future possible, a vision of the future has to be sold, even if it is a vision that will never be realized" (Rajan 2017: 115–16). This is similarly the case in the marketing campaigns directed at egg freezing (positioned as "fertility preservation" or extending fertility) in which the ability to freeze for a potential future is animated yet also contradictory due to the fact that only a small group of women return to the clinic to use their frozen gametes, for example.[3] Consequently, biocapital (or what here may be referred to as cryo-capital) relies on a promissory rhetoric as well as a particular temporal logic. Both elements are related to the making of value: "Vision, hype, speculation, and temporality all relate to questions of value" (Rajan 2017: 116).

How best to handle reproductive waste is a highly sensitive matter. In what Thompson (2005) refers to as the biomedical mode of reproduction, she delineates how reproductive matter becomes promissory as well as profane. To Thompson (2005), reproductive waste is not exclusively a logistical problem. Rather, it becomes an ethical and a gendered problem conceptualized as a balance between "the sacred life potential and profane material aspects of the body tissues and treatment prerogatives. A rupture in any of these paths potentially involves alienation of the body from the person" (Thompson 2005: 256). When seen as sacred, biological matter (the embryo, for example) is treated carefully in light of its promissory value, while when unsuccessful (an egg cell that does not develop, for example), biological matter may more readily enter other economies such as the stem cell industry. In reference to a talk presented by Charis Thompson, Kietzer (2012) notes that this circulation is additionally gendered. In her presentation titled "Three Times a Woman," Thompson (2012) pinpoints how women, in the story of Proposition 71 in California,[4] were differentially invested in the fertility industry: women were voters for Prop 71, they were producers of what became labeled as "IVF by-products" (egg cells, placentas, urine), and finally, women, in the story of Proposition 71, became positioned as consumers of products tied to the stem cell industry (anti-aging cosmetics, for example). This is similarly the case with placenta donations in the European and Asian context in which women frequently handle the material, donate the material, and later consume the material.

Following in the footsteps of scholars like Rajan (2017) and Thompson (2005), this book brings culture into the analysis of reproductive waste and value. It prioritizes the exchanges that take place between waste and value, and thus, views reproductive donations as objects "in transit" (Moster 2002: 93). Similarly to Moster (2002), I stress that waste and culture are entangled practices. This is readily the case with reproductive donations that exist both inside and outside the body. When inside the body, these donations are "naturally" in place and so have a particular value. Once outside the body—either because they are extracted or "naturally" expelled—they become potential sources of impurity, or even hazardous waste that is best whisked away and discarded. To this extent, reproductive donations exist in the uncomfortable zone between the home/market, the private/public, value/dignity, and subject/object (Roberts 2012). The processes involved in the extraction and insertion of human ova, for example, necessitate removing what may have the appearance of something private (and perhaps even sacred in some cultural contexts) and repositioning it (intelligent, young, white, tall, healthy eggs, for example) in a market economy. This is also the case in terms of placenta donation. Here the placenta may be framed as a sibling to the newborn baby or as the baby's first home, making donation an intimate, personal matter to render the placenta's transition into a commodity less morally suspect.

So how do reproductive donations gain value? To respond to this question, I also draw on the concept of biovalue developed by Catherine Waldby (2000). According to Waldby (2000), blood, tissue, and DNA are productive in generating economic value. To her, biovalue involves a transformation and potential enhancement of biological matter: "Biovalue is generated wherever the generative and transformative productivity of living entities can be instrumentalized along lines which make them useful for human projects—science, industry, medicine, agriculture or other arenas of technical culture" (Waldby 2000: 33). It is tissue with potential value. Whereas scientific advancements give bio-objects new life, the productivity of various bio-objects draws upon transnational market economies as well (Waldby and Mitchell 2006). Moreover, the concept of biovalue is relevant in discussing the affective economies involved in biomedical advancements. Novas (2006) illustrates this swiftly in his analyses of bio-objects that are turned into valuable biomedical products within patient organizations, through an affective economy involving desire and hope. Similarly, Bharadwaj and Glasner (2009) situate the biovalue of stem cell therapies as promissory—exchanging capital and hope for speculative treatments.

Biomedical infrastructures have paved the way for bio-objects to gain new value through processes of recycling and the reinstatement of certain bodies as bioavailable and supplementary (Bharadwaj 2012; Cohen 2004). In the global politics of body parts and reproductive waste, the bodies from the Global South, in particular women's and poor people's bodies and parts, are made to appear bioavailable (chapter 5). Hair is recycled from haircutting salons to the wig and hair extension industry, organs are removed and transplanted into other bodies, bones are turned into ritual instruments or skeletons on display in various anatomy classes, and recently human stool has been finding new value as fecal microbiota transplants, a process in which a provider's stool is mixed with a saline solution and placed in another patient for the purpose of boosting the patient's own good bacteria.

Having briefly outlined theoretical perspectives and key concepts on reproductive waste and value, I now turn to a discussion of how reproductive donations, along with the ideas and imaginations, enter local/global discourses and practices.

On Globalization and Mobility

In conceptualizing reproductive donations as global and mobile, I turn to feminist scholars who note that globalization is neither a stable nor a singular force, but one that is frequently stratified, contradictory, and partial (Bharadwaj and Glasner 2009; Colen 1995;

Franklin et al. 2000; Lash and Lury 2001; Strathern 1991). To Franklin et al., the global is repeatedly transfigured, a fantasy, a set of situated practices conceptualized, for instance, in the global icons of the blue planet, the fetus, and the cell (Franklin et al. 2000: 5). Focusing on the politics of stratified reproductive labor, Vora (2015) situates global reproduction critically as a type of vital energy or life support readily made available and accessible through postcolonial infrastructures and pathways. Similarly, in their analysis of embryonic stem cell research in India, Bharadwaj and Glasner problematize the global/local as no longer "bounded sites" (Bharadwaj and Glasner 2009: 5) but paths through which ideas, imagination, resources, technologies, people, matter, and capital travel. Consequently, to Bharadwaj and Glasner (2009), the idea of the global/local has become "shaken up" and dislocated. Throughout this book, *the global* additionally functions as an analytical device—a discursive condition, as well as a set of material practices—while *mobility* is used to discuss the ways that reproductive fluids flow as well as the ways that practices frequently are embedded within neoliberal and neocolonial understandings of the female reproductive body.

Global Reproduction

The recognition that reproduction and globalization intersect is by no means new (Inhorn 2010, 2011, 2015; Inhorn and Shrivastav 2010; Kroløkke et al. 2012; Vora 2015). Inhorn (2010) has already theorized how reproductive objects, patients, and technologies move across nation-states. In her research centering the UAE and Dubai, Inhorn (2015) brings the notion of cosmopolitan medicine in dialogue with empirical research on fertility travel. In the practice of what becomes described as "global gynecology" (Inhorn 2015: 40), Dubai is situated as a cosmopolitan fertility or reprohub characterized by a combination of tradition (its roots as a former trading hub) and contemporary allure (a popular shopping and tourism destination). The dynamics of globalized reproduction are similarly present in the development of the concept of reproscapes (Inhorn and Shrivastav 2010). The concept of reproscapes is used to underscore the complex interrelationship that unfolds when technologies, bodies, body parts, money, and desire become situated within the context of fertility travel, for example:

> Reproductive tourism occurs in a new world order, characterized not only by circulating reproductive technologies (technoscapes), but also by circulating reproductive actors (ethnoscapes) and their body parts

> (bioscapes), leading to a large-scale global industry (financescapes), in which images (mediascapes) and ideas (ideoscapes) about making lovely babies while "on holiday" come into play. Furthermore, this reproscape is highly gendered—with technologies enacted on men's and women's bodies in highly differentiated ways. (Inhorn and Shrivastav 2010: 69S)

Clearly, the notion of reproscapes advances an interesting theoretical perspective on globalization, including how we come to understand kinship in a time when bodies, biogenetic substances, media images, money, and clinical expertise cross borders and create new contexts for imagining and making relatedness. It is less explicit, however, in providing the analyst with a critical toolbox on how globalized reproduction frequently gets contextualized within a set of neoliberal and neocolonial practices. For example, what may be referred to as "fertility consumers" tend to consist of individuals from the Global North who enterprise-up for better and younger cells and go global to fulfill their dreams of parenting (Kroløkke 2009). Inhorn recognizes this when she makes reference to reproscapes as stratified, however: "The adjective *stratified* might be added to the term *reproscape* to describe the inequalities, disjunctures, and obstacles that inhibit and even prevent flows of people, technology, and other forms across uneven global terrains" (Inhorn 2015: 24). Not only are reproscapes gendered, they also reveal that global reproduction is uneven, at times available only to some.

Feminist scholars reiterate this more critical perspective on global reproduction and situate it within neoliberal ideology and neocolonialism (Cohen 2004; Scheper-Hughes 2000; Vora 2015). Here, the global market in reproduction is similarly stratified (Colen 1995), while neoliberal ideology revamps women into (good) active reproductive citizens. Within neoliberal ideology, individuals are seen as individually responsible for taking care of their fertility (Kroløkke and Pant 2012). The attention to neoliberalism is similarly visible in Vora's (2015) work on surrogacy in India. According to her, the outsourcing of reproductive labor to India is entangled with a postcolonial logic in which low earning is made to appear civilized and gestational surrogacy turned potentially empowering, when surrogates enter into "property relations to their bodies and a sense of entrepreneurship of themselves" (Vora 2015: 11). In this set of research, globalized reproduction is inextricably tied to historically, gendered, and racial structures embedded within North-South relations.

Reproduction is, as noted in feminist scholarship, global in another sense as well. In vitro fertilization (IVF) has been essential in the creation of innovative and globalized biomedical platforms (Franklin 2013). To Franklin (2013), IVF has been at the foundation of the other innovative and global biological platforms, such as those found within regenerative medicine (stem cells, for example) and in the spatial construction of IVF/stem cell laboratories in which eggs and embryos can easily pass in and out of the promise of life and the promise of health. The technological platform of IVF has, she notes, been driven not exclusively out of a desire for children but largely by economics. As echoed in financial accounts, IVF is entangled in the market in petri dishes, laboratory equipment, gametes, and fertility hormones collectively constituting a globally growing industry (Toft 2015). As noted by Franklin, "These biotranslational fields are, like IVF, driven not only by research priorities but by economics" (Franklin 2013: 38).

While IVF has contributed to what is here referred to as the making of global innovation platforms in reproduction and health, localized reproductive donations are made into globalized bioproducts that turn the consumption of someone else's nature acceptable and even desirable. This is evident in Franklin's (2013) historical account of IVF as well as in the empirical accounts of infertile Danish women traveling to Spain for oocyte donation (Kroløkke 2014). In these accounts, gamete donation is narrated as borrowing (not purchasing) someone else's fertility (Kroløkke 2014; Nahman 2013, 2011, 2008). At the same time, egg providers from different geographical locations travel across national borders to give, they say, a necessary "baking ingredient" and the "gift of motherhood" (Kroløkke 2015). In this manner, intending parents as well as egg providers, along with various clinical actors (medical personnel, for example) and technologies, escape the market yet turn reproductive matter into globalized bio-objects that "naturally" (and easily) cross reproductive paths between differently situated women.

Theorizing this globalized market in reproduction and health, Bharadwaj and Glasner's concept of biocrossing is particularly apt at showing how ideas, as well as people, technologies, and matter, move across physical borders, between biology and machine, and across different ethical domains: "A bio-crossing is conceptualized as a passage or crossing that traverses the borders of biology, moves between biology and machine, and passes across geo-political, commercial, ethical and moral borders" (Bharadwaj and Glasner 2009: 7). Whereas Bharadwaj and Glasner (2009) focus on stem cell research and bio-crossings undertaken in India, the concept of bio-crossing shows how mobility is contingent upon the availability of provider bodies, clinical infrastructures, transportation, medical visas, terminally ill patients, and also medical clinicians capable and willing to perform particular procedures. As noted by Cohen (2004), in his formulation of bioavailable bodies, and further supported by Scheper-Hughes (2000) in her work on organ transplants, bodies without future (frequently poor, dark-skinned, female bodies) are positioned as waste and are consequently made to appear available in the global market in human body parts and reproductive services.

Global reproduction not only translates into other platforms but also serves as a crossover to other medical platforms, disrupting human-animal crossings in the process. Notably, human reproductive science has historically benefited from a close relationship to developments within the animal reproductive sciences (Franklin 2007; Thompson 2011; Svendsen 2014). Svendsen (2014) delineates this relationship in her analysis of Danish piglets and premature infants in the neonatal unit in Copenhagen. According to her, "Reproductive and perinatal science is populated with animals made viable and killable to develop reproductive technologies and create life for human infants" (Svendsen 2014: 183). Deeply entangled with research ambitions in the development of regenerative medicine intended for humans, animals become, as Thompson (2011) shows, boundary figures. This is notably the case with Dolly the Sheep, who became an "animal model for a technique that has become one of the basic elements in the production of new markets and products that belong to a new form of capital" (Franklin 2007: 117). It is similarly the case when the scarcity of human female eggs is combined with the proposal to use cow eggs in the development of patient-specific embryonic stem cell lines (Thompson 2011: 203). As these examples show, IVF is intertwined with regenerative medicine, creating "new kinds of biological connections" (Franklin 2013: 38) as well as the potential for new human/animal biomedical products: "Some of these products are 'purely' human; others are from every species imaginable, but most of them are of mixed genealogical and technological ancestry" (Franklin 2013: 38).

Animals have far exceeded their value as stand-ins or "ethical replacements" (Thompson 2011: 193) for human life. They are also symbols of scientific progress and have become embedded in notions of nationhood (Franklin 2007). For example, the world's first cloned dog—Snuppy (the "Seoul National University puppy")—became an emblem of South Korean research achievements (Thompson 2011), while in Singapore the tropical zebra fish contributed to the country's establishment as an international fish farming research environment (Thompson 2011: 131–34). Similarly, the sheep (and Dolly the Sheep in particular) became interwoven with British notions of prosperity and nationhood (Franklin 2007), while in Denmark all parts of the pig, including its meat, (potentially) semen, bones, skin, and (potentially) placenta, constitute valuable export commodities and contribute financially to the making of the Danish welfare state (Svendsen 2014: 182). Whether as research participants or export commodities, animals as boundary figures play a vital role in the tying of agricultural pasts with international research hubs and the development of reproductive techniques ultimately available to humans as well.

In these various entanglements, reproductive donations take up a set of globalizing qualities. Transgressing countries and organizational settings, reproductive donations become material, affective, and discursive (Nahman 2006), sometimes even crossing the lines between humans and animals and, as already noted, between reproductive and regenerative medicine. Reproductive objects are, similar to in Lash and Lury's (2007) scholarship on the culture industries, throughout the book, viewed as objects that come into existence through a set of discursive, affective, organizational, and material relations. Reproductive donations are local in the sense that they come from particular women's bodies and are consumed by other individual women. However, they are also globalized as they leave individual bodies and enter clinics, laboratories, freezers, pickup trucks, factories, countries, for example. Additionally, they are made to appear global in the sense that they are constructed as "naturally" moving across national borders: urine is donated in the Netherlands and collected, processed, and sold as hormonal medication throughout Europe, while oocytes in Greece are exchanged for cash, extracted, cryopreserved, and shipped to locations worldwide. Thus, throughout this book, globalized reproduction is a key theoretical as well as analytical concept. As noted by Lash and Lury, this understanding of globalization does not position objects as either simply global or local but rather as "temporal, rhythmic morphologies" (Lash and Lury 2007: 19) that move in and out of globality.

Mobile Fluids

Reproductive substances are not only global; they are also made to appear mobile. To Inhorn (2015), the concept of reproductive flows captures the fluid qualities of reproductive bodies (patients, clinicians, gamete providers), substances (hormones, gametes, menstruation, embryos), and technologies (petri dishes and IVF techniques that move from site to site). The concept of Reproflow privileges the movements that appear within each of the aforementioned reproscapes while also noting that bodily flows are, at times, blocked or—due to economic resources, laws, availability, reproductive access, cultural barriers, quality, or long waiting lists—simply difficult at best (Inhorn 2015: 26–27). Thus, while Shenfield et al. (2010) estimate that a minimum of twenty-four to thirty thousand cycles of cross-border fertility treatments could be taking place each year throughout Europe involving eleven to fourteen thousand patients, this considerable flow of patients crossing European national borders produces not only new babies but also new ethical and legal concerns related to the rights and availability of reproductive services (Shenfield et al. 2010). In each of the case study chapters that follow, I return to a discussion of the mobility constraints pertaining to the ways that urine, oocytes, and placentas flow.

Mobility concerns not only the ways that fluids flow (or are blocked from flowing) but also the ways that reproductive fluids mobilize particular understandings of the reproductive body. For example, oocytes from Spanish women mobilize an understanding of gift-giving provider bodies while oocytes from Russian women, from the perspective of Danish interviewees, conjure up concerns related to reproductive trafficking (Kroløkke 2014). Moreover, reproductive fluids mobilize different understandings and follow different trajectories. They are biological in some instances (fluids deprived of identity and social relations, such as the porcine placenta that is transported from Denmark to Japan) but become, as defined by Svendsen (2014), biographical in other contexts (situated in a loving relationship, such as when the human placenta is recognized as baby's first home). Whereas Svendsen uses this distinction in her research to discuss how (some) premature infants or piglets become biographical creatures, it, jointly with the connection to temporality (fluids with a past, a present, as well as a future), has obvious relevance to the ways that the reproductive fluids in this book are mobilized. Biographical life is characterized, as noted by Svendsen, by a past and present life that, in particular contexts, also bears hope and future potentiality (Svendsen 2014: 188). Taking this perspective to heart methodologically implies attention to how reproductive fluids move as well as also how the context itself is mobilized and performed (Lie and Lykke 2017; Sheller and Urry 2006). As will become evident throughout the book, reproductive fluids transition and transform in very localized contexts (Kopytoff 1986).

Mobility is always contingent. In the case of oocytes, for example, mobility depends on available young and fertile women, reproductive work (hormone intake, extraction techniques, psychological counseling), as well as clinical spaces, pain medication, ultrasound machines, petri dishes and freezing containers, in addition to mobility becoming materialized in very specific, localized acts. Oocytes may move across national borders as well as compensation rules, recognition, technologies, and clinical success rates. Once oocytes leave the body in these enactments, they become imaginary constructs that are frequently narrated as altruistic gifts, surplus material, waste, biocapital, or, in the case of elective freezing, they mobilize feelings of relief as they become re-articulated as an investment in the future, for example (see figure 1.1.). I argue that these cultural and social narratives enable other movements to unfold. When oocytes are mobilized as gifts or surplus material, their movements are more "naturally" directed to the fertility clinic. In contrast, when mobilized as waste by the fertility industry, they more readily enter

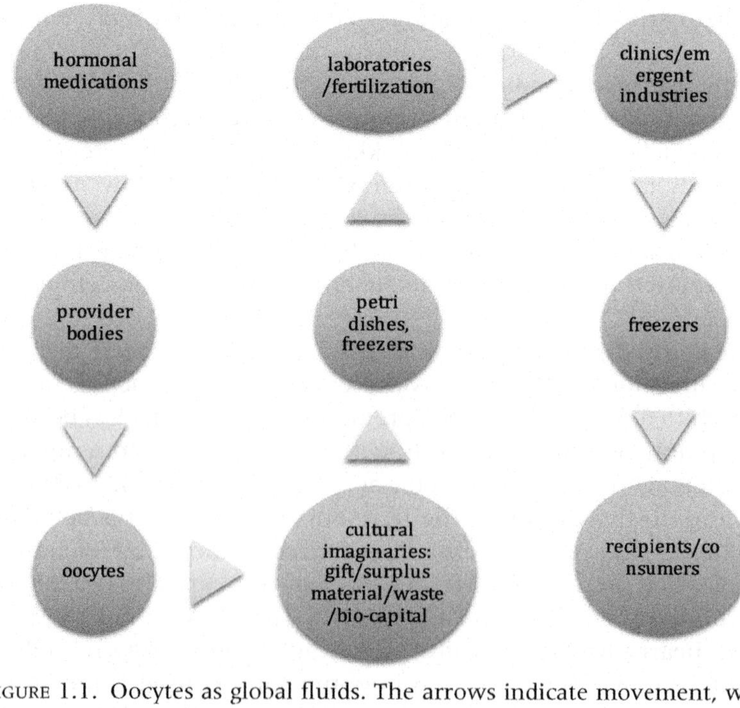

Figure 1.1. Oocytes as global fluids. The arrows indicate movement, while the circles indicate a temporary stasis of sorts.

into emergent industries, such as the stem cell industry; when mobilized as a future investment, they are stored in freezers located at various biobanks.

The above visualization of oocytes as global fluids cements the idea that mobility is contingent upon a number of factors. The ways in which oocytes move are predicated on hormonal medications, reproductive work, female and fertile bodies, extraction techniques, cryopreservation media, cultural imaginaries (waste, surplus material, gifts, biocapital, and future investment), a legal framework that similarly enables oocytes to move or remain inactive (as cryopreserved parts), clinical expertise, petri dishes, freezers, laboratory equipment and recipients/consumers. Mobility can then be framed as involving (a) the transfer and exchange of reproductive substances between differently situated bodies (in the case of providing oocytes between differently situated women), (b) different industrial and clinical practices that enable mobility to unfold, (c) the ways in which new media communication environments facilitate a form of virtual travel and engage relational geographies,[5] and (d) the ways in which reproductive donations engage different cultural values and imaginations, as made manifest when oocytes are framed as gifts, surplus material, biocapital, investments, or waste. Tracking reproductive donations grant me an enhanced understanding of the lifespan of each donation.

In the case of placentas, mobility involves birthing bodies, afterbirth matter, hospital settings, bags, doctors/midwives/nurses, containers, pickup vans, drivers, industrial processes, money, and global branding strategies. Dripping with blood, the placenta exits the body as afterbirth matter. Typically, within the Western medical science context, the healthcare provider (such as the obstetrician or the midwife) first examines the placenta and then puts it into a hospital bin or a bowl, forwarding it either to a laboratory for testing and/or disposing of it as biohazard waste. Not depicted in figure 1.2 is the recent trend within the more modern natural, holistic, and midwifery approaches: women bringing the placenta home and turning it into herbal remedies. After the placenta is delivered and held, perhaps even handled, examined, or photographed by family members, it is cooked, blended, or dehydrated and then consumed as afterbirth nutrients (as pills or smoothies, for example). Presented in the figure below is the emergence of placentas as medical injections, cosmetics, anti-aging creams, whitening lotions, and other beauty products. From waste to considerable personal, cultural, and medical significance, the human as well as animal placenta moves

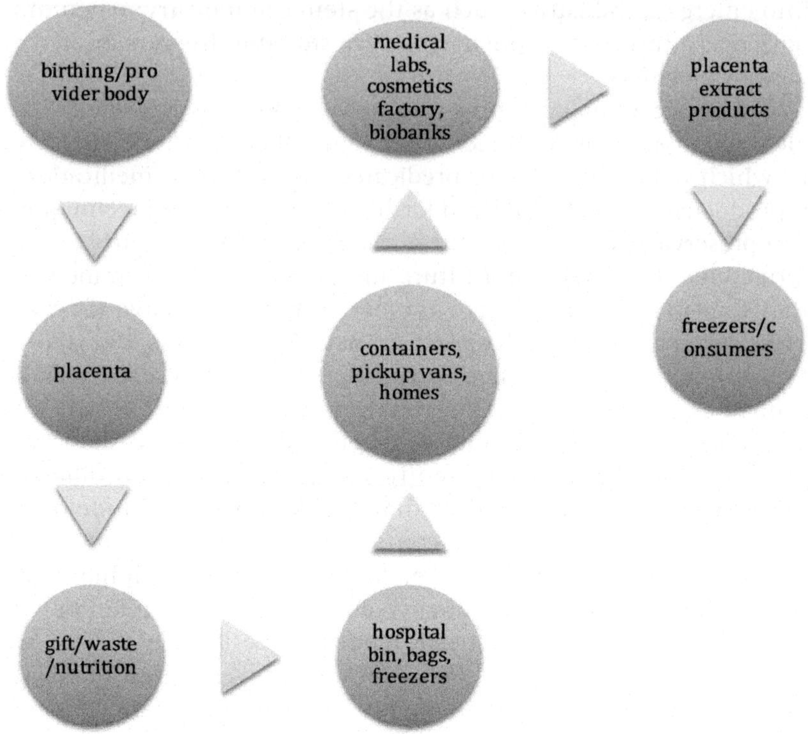

FIGURE 1.2. Placenta as global fluid. The arrows indicate movement, while the circles indicate inactivity or stasis, however temporary.

through the exchange processes that are constructed to meet various consumptive needs.

The movements and stasis involved in urine donation appear at first glance to be less complex. Urine donation in the Netherlands is built upon the fact that pregnant women produce urine on a regular basis. Within a rhetorical trope of sister solidarity, Dutch pregnant women are encouraged to sign up as donors or urine providers. The provider then self-administers and collects her urine from the sixth to the sixteenth week of pregnancy, during which time she produces the most hormones. She leaves it outside her door in containers ready to be picked up by drivers hired by the organization Moeders voor Moeders (Mothers for Mothers). The urine is transported to the Dutch factory and turned into fertility hormone medication and human chorionic gonadotropin (hCG) pregnancy test kits. While urine most profoundly exemplifies (reproductive) waste, it is reframed as a form of gifting when situated in a donation practice, while within

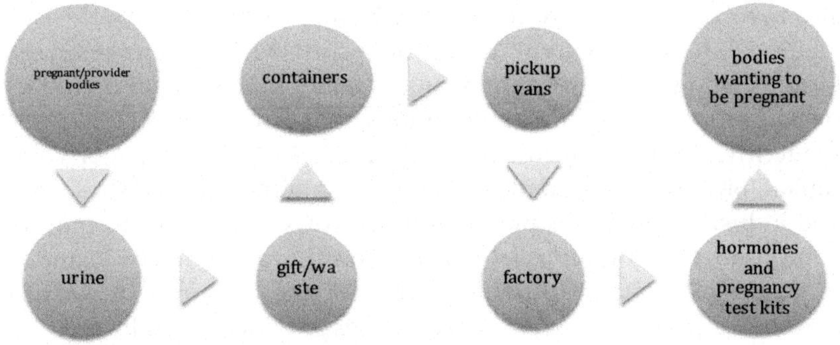

FIGURE 1.3. Urine as global fluid. The arrows indicate movement, while the circles indicate stasis, however temporary.

the context of pregnancy it is also a marker of a healthy pregnancy. In return for their work in the donation program, Dutch urine donors receive a bracelet as a token of appreciation.

The above visual depictions, along with the existing feminist research, illustrate that reproductive donations take on different and at times contradictory meanings (Gupta and Richters 2008; Santoro 2011). In this book I track the ways in which reproductive donations circulate and entangle to become different bioproducts. In choosing to view reproductive donations as *entangled,* I draw upon the notion that legal, ethical, cultural, technological, bodily relations, and clinical practices are intertwined. When employed analytically, entanglement, as well as the accompanying terms of dis- and re-entanglement, conceptualize how reproductive tissue, gametes, and embryos move in clinical practices, in and out of freezing tanks and IVF laboratories, between bodies, from IVF clinics to stem cell laboratories, in cultural imaginations, and in marketization processes (Callon 1998). Reproductive donations are simultaneously located in particular kin relations; cultural and affective economies of hope, uncertainty, potentiality, fear (Ahmed 2004; 2010; Franklin 2013); as well as the geopolitical inequalities in which global reproduction benefits individuals differently (Cohen 2004).

Throughout this book I stress the complexities involved when oocytes, placentas, and urine obtain globalizing and mobilizing qualities. They involve biological matter, images, paperwork, contracts, medications, law, money, technologies, love, hope, and desire that jointly move or facilitate movement. Thus, positioning reproductive donations as global not only entails studying how biogenetic substances circulate transnationally to become global bioproducts, but it also involves other reproductive actors such as legislators, ethicists, medical experts, new communication technologies, medical experts, farmers, and freezing and thawing capacities that are vital in understanding how reproductive donations move transnationally. Consequently, I argue that imagination, legislation, affects, paperwork, capital, physical equipment (e.g. boxes, containers, petri dishes, etc.) and industrial processes play important roles in the transformation of reproductive donations from waste to value and must be included to gain a more holistic understanding of the dynamics at stake. I emphasize concrete practices and settings in which reproductive donations are performed, positioned, and enacted. Additionally, I note how cultural and frequently conventional ideas of waste and bioavailable bodies play an important role in positioning reproductive matter at different parts of its lifespan, as legitimately moving into the circuit of scientific and commercial exchanges. And I follow a more biographical approach delineated by Lash and Lury (2001) in their work on cultural commodities, when I ask: What are the key components of the ways in which reproductive donations move? Who are the key actors? What are the key moments? How is the reproductive donation transformed from context to context?

Conclusion

This chapter outlined feminist cultural analytical perspectives on the ways that rhetorical strategies, metaphors, affects of love and desire, along with specific material "things" and sensory landscapes, come together to form particular understandings of the reproductive body. Feminist cultural analysis illustrates how global fluids move from one reproductive universe (e.g., procreation or waste) to another (e.g., science and commodification). The analytical framework was presented as a tool that helps deconstruct the ways in which rhetoric, communication, affects, and matter come together and constitute particular understandings of reproductive donations—oocytes, placentas, and urine. Different rhetorical, affective, and material constructions of reproductive donations produce different moral concerns and strategies for action (concluding chapter). The concepts of global fluids and reproductive mobility were used to discuss the ways in which reproductive matter, laws, affects, money, technologies, and expertise circulate and achieve a certain level of fluidity. Global fluids are reinvented and re-naturalized as particular bioproducts. Globalization erodes boundaries of time and space, giving rise to tensions between social, biological, legal, ethical, and genetic understandings of parenthood as well as between values and economic interests. In this manner national boundaries are transgressed, reproduction is commercialized, some bodies become biological resources or are made to appear bioavailable, and nations find new ways to police the ways that reproductive fluids may flow.

Notes

1. Recycle Yourself, http://gorecycleyourself.com/ (retrieved February 2016) illustrates this type of rhetoric. The website encourages its viewers to consider becoming organ donors.
2. More can be read at Recycle Yourself, "Donation Stories," http://gorecycleyourself.com/about-donation/donation-stories.php (retrieved February 2016).
3. According to an Australian survey of one hundred women who froze their eggs between 1999 and 2014, only 6 percent of them returned to use their egg cells and 3 percent of them were successful in achieving a live birth: X. Pham, "How Many Women Actually Use Their Frozen Eggs?," Labroots, 22 January 2017, https://www.labroots.com/trending/clinical-and-molecular-dx/5109/women-use-frozen-eggs (retrieved September 2017).
4. Proposition 71 was passed in California in 2004, making stem cell research a constitutional right. California's stem cell agency was created as a result, with a specific goal to advance the field of regenerative medicine. More information can be found at the agency's website: https://www.cirm.ca.gov/about-cirm/history (retrieved September 2017).
5. This is seen, for example, when Spanish clinics in their online marketing material use the image of a friendly Spain to situate Spanish donors as "natural" gift-giving young women (Kroløkke 2014).

Chapter 2

URINE

FROM WASTE TO HORMONE SHOTS

"I will happily send you a bottle of urine for some tulips," a pregnant colleague of mine, located in the United States, told me when I embarked on my first trip to the Netherlands to visit the Moeders voor Moeders (Mothers for Mothers, MvM) organization and the pharmaceutical company Aspen Oss. MvM collects urine from pregnant Dutch women, which Aspen Oss then processes into an active ingredient sold to the pharmaceutical company Merck Sharp & Dohme (MSD).[1] MSD packages and sells the active ingredient as the drug Pregnyl, which is aimed at women undergoing IVF treatment, although the product can also be used in cases of young boys whose testicles have failed to drop down naturally into their scrotum and also, notably without the approval of the company, as a slimming drug used in the weight-loss industry. In this chapter, I first locate urine donation within a larger "peecycling" movement, and I show how ideas on reproductive waste play an integral role in the collection and recirculation of urine. Throughout the chapter, I focus on the components that enable urine to move, interrogating how urine and also affects and practices with urine are transformed from context to context. I argue that it is precisely urine's ontological status as "waste" that enables its potentiality (for example, as hormone medication or fertilizer). When coupled with what has the appearance of a naturalized desire for motherhood, urine recirculates into the Dutch fertility industry and beyond, through a collective ethos of patriotic solidarity and sisterhood.

Urine Sites

Urine is big business.[2] Beyond the IVF industry, the Rich Earth Institute, located in the United States, advocates recycling human urine and using it as a fertilizer in the agricultural industry. According to the Rich Earth Institute, urine can be collected and transported "odorlessly,"[3] and because it is rich in phosphorus—a mineral needed in the fertilizing of plants—it can be turned into sanitized and sustainable fertilizer. An adult urine provider produces enough urine (100–150 gallons a year) to fertilize enough grain to produce a daily loaf of bread.[4] The institute argues that urine-diverting toilets could enable the production of cheap and necessary fertilizer and additionally contribute to the successful conservation of water, leading to a reduction in wastewater treatment costs. In the promotional material, a young, friendly (smiling) white male, situated in a green lush forest area, stands on top of a white, clean-looking pickup truck next to a sizable blue container (presumably his contribution). The image makes urine donation appear easy, even pleasant. Amsterdam's water utility, Waternet, had similar ambitions when, during the International Water Week held in Amsterdam in 2013, they installed temporary public urinals (men only) in the city to help harvest pee, now labeled "green urine," intended for use in the fertilization of Amsterdam's rooftop gardens.[5] In a different but nevertheless related manner, the drinking of one's own urine is seen as a health act by the Urine Therapy Association based in Hong Kong. Here, urine is framed as alternative medicine that helps the body recuperate and regain its former strength. What may have the appearance of being a smelly and unattractive fluid exiting the body as a waste product has been newly presented in a discourse of sustainability, health, and "liquid gold" in the MvM recruitment material and online urine provider stories.[6]

The empirical material that has gone into this urine assemblage has primarily been obtained from one case study: the MvM organization, located in the Netherlands.[7] I made two visits to the Netherlands, which included a visit to the organization, interviews with MvM employees, and reviews of marketing and recruitment material, urine provider experiences, and stories displayed on the organization's website, as well as on online forums, and vlogs and photos made available by MvM from its historical archive. Briefly, MvM is a nationwide organization in the Netherlands whose headquarters is located in the small town of Oss, approximately a two-hour train ride from Amsterdam. Oss is in the industrial heart of the Netherlands. It is a town of approximately sixty thousand inhabitants, and with the visible presence of pharmaceutical companies and factories it has a strong blue-collar feel. MvM is physically located next to two major pharmaceutical companies in Oss, and although it is a separate organization, MvM is owned by Aspen Oss (formerly Organon and Merck & Co),[8] a pharmaceutical company with a long history of turning waste products into active ingredients in the making of pharmaceutical products. Aside from the development of the active ingredient (pregnant women's urine) needed in the production of Pregnyl, Aspen Oss is also known for isolating and developing the active ingredient in animal pancreas needed for insulin. Since 1931, MvM has specialized in the development of human chorionic gonadotropin (hCG), exclusively based on pregnant women's urine. Approximately thirty-five thousand women donate annually in the Netherlands, producing close to 1.3 million liters of urine a year.[9] Providers are recruited through word of mouth, a strong online presence, a carefully developed website, and Facebook. During my second trip to the Netherlands, I arrived in the midst of MvM's eighty-fifth birthday celebrations, which depicted MvM as an intergenerational Dutch success story, tying the previous donations of older women together with the current donations of younger, pregnant women.

To become a urine provider, a pregnant woman must donate her urine between the sixth and sixteenth week of pregnancy. While donations are freely and altruistically provided to MvM, each provider receives a small and token gift package from the organization. Not everyone can be a provider. The prospective provider has to affirm her health by responding to a series of questions that are asked of blood donors as well. The following criteria limit potential donors: women who have received a blood transfusion after 1 January 1980; have spent a total of six months or more in the United Kingdom between 1 January 1980 and 31 December 1996; or have HIV cannot become urine providers. Similar to blood donation and what Copeman calls "hemato-global assemblages" (Copeman 2009: 2), urine providing relies upon a particular set of standards and protocols. The provider agrees to gather her daily urine in blue containers and places the bottles in an agreed-upon spot, making them available for discreet, MvM promises, weekly pickups. Once delivered to the factory, urine undergoes several procedures. Because urine is the necessary active ingredient in Pregnyl and the demand for Pregnyl is ever increasing, MvM is looking to expand its urine base. This involves recruiting new providers (the thirty-five thousand providers constitute approximately 20 percent of pregnant Dutch women who are providers on an annual basis) or optimizing an already existing provider group through the development of mobile collection bags or an MvM toilet specially designed for urine collection. In this way, urine providing is not only available to all pregnant women as an altruistic donation practice, but, because not all pregnant women are permitted to donate, it is simultaneously also a practice that "re-inscribes the boundaries of civic belonging and exclusion," as echoed by Valentine in her analysis of blood donation (Valentine 2005: 117). Having briefly introduced MvM as the chapter's main case study, I turn now to the development of hCG and the ways that urine has emerged as a global fluid.

The Emergence of hCG and Urine Donation

The choice to use urine in the development of fertility hormones is not new. Nevertheless, what made women's urine the right choice for making the IVF drug Pregnyl? In her book titled *Beyond the Natural Body: An Archeology of Sex Hormones,* Oudshoorn (1994) convincingly traces the discovery of urine as a potent force in the production of sex hormones. As recounted by Oudshoorn (1994), the discovery involved the joint work and ambitions of gynecologists, laboratory scientists, pharmaceutical companies, pregnant and postmenopausal women, and slaughterhouses. As she notes, this time with specific reference to the use of human urine, "The actors had to rely on the gynecologists: scientists could only obtain the urine of pregnant women from gynecological clinics. This became a new source of inexpensive and easily available material for research on female sex hormones, and signaled the end of the period in which research was constrained by the scarcity of research material" (Oudshoorn 1994: 73). In this section, I build on Lunenfeld (2004) and Oudshoorn's (1994) work, supplementing it with information gained from visits to and interviews at MvM, to contextualize the development of hCG.

After the discovery that women's urine contained gonadotropic hormones—proven to stimulate follicular growth—scientists first developed and used the hormones in animal experiments (Lunenfeld 2004). Whereas researchers discovered that pregnant women's urine contained the placenta-based hormone used in the production of hCG, the urine of post-menopausal women, according to Tausk, contained the material needed in the production of follicle stimulating hormone (FSH) and luteinizing hormone (LH), referred to as HMG (human menopausal gonadotropin) (Tausk 1975: 122). As scientists determined that middle-aged women's urine contained hCG or HMG, it led to more systematic urine collection efforts. In the 1950s, human menopausal urine was regularly collected in four main centers, located respectively in the Netherlands, Spain, Italy, and Israel (Lunenfeld 2004). The collected urine was then used in the extraction of HMG, and, in the case of the Netherlands, hCG was extracted from pregnant women's urine used in the production of Pregnyl.

According to Lunenfeld (2004), human pituitaries and menopausal urine were the sole sources for the extraction and production of HMG for years, but since the mid-1990s, this has been challenged in several ways. For one, the four above-mentioned urine centers were unable to provide enough urine to an ever-growing market (Lunenfeld 2004). Whereas early on the centers relied on a total of 600 pregnant and postmenopausal women as urine providers, contributing 120,000 liters of urine a year, Lunenfeld (2004) argues that today a whopping 120 million liters would be necessary to satisfy the demand, leading to a requirement for approximately 600,000 providers. As a direct result of the need for more urine in the field of human and also animal reproduction, collection centers were outsourced from the mid-1970s to the 1990s in locales such as Korea, China, India, and Brazil, enabling access to larger bioavailable populations. However, the development of centers outside Europe led to concerns about regulatory control, quality, and safety (Lunenfeld 2004). The need for a constant and reliable supply of urine therefore encouraged researchers to develop laboratory-based hormone products (Lunenfeld 2004). While more reliable in terms of general quality, these products are also more expensive. Accordingly, MvM has played a stabilizing role, and today the organization continues to use pregnant women's urine as its sole source of urine supply, employing many of the same processing facilities in Oss and Boxtel that were used in the early part of the company's history.

Little is known about the first four European urine centers. The development of follicle stimulating hormones is, however, partially attributed to the work undertaken in one of the centers—the pharmaceutical company Serono, then based in Italy—and the donation of urine is known to have been undertaken by Roman Catholic nuns. While the vice president of Serono is said to have positioned urine donation as similar to blood donation (Birrittieri 2005), it appears

PREGNYL:	MENOPUR:
(Human Chorionic Gonadotropin) INFORMATION FOR THE DOCTOR 1. NAME OF THE MEDICINAL PRODUCT Pregnyl ® 5000 I.U. powder for solution for injection. 2. QUALITATIVE AND QUANTITATIVE COMPOSITION Pregnyl consists of a freeze-dried powder for injection. The active ingredient [human chorionic gonadotropin (hCG)], which is obtained from the urine of pregnant women, has luteinizing hormone (LH) activity. An ampoule contains 5,000 I.U. hCG.	Menopur injection contains human menopausal gonadotropin (sometimes known as menotropin) as the active ingredient. Human menopausal gonadotropin is a combination of two naturally occurring female hormones—follicle stimulating hormone (FSH) and luteinizing hormone (LH)—extracted and purified from the urine of postmenopausal women. It is used in the treatment of infertility. FSH and LH directly affect the ovaries in women and the testicles in men.
Source: https://www.medicines.org.uk/emc/medicine/12613 Retrieved September 2016	Source: http://www.netdoctor.co.uk/medicines/pregnancy/a7077/menopur-human-menopausal-gonadotrophin/ Retrieved September 2016.

FIGURES 2.1 and 2.2. Descriptions of the ingredients of Pregnyl and Menopur. Whereas the active ingredient in Pregnyl is hCG derived from the urine of pregnant women, the active ingredient in Menopur is human menopausal gonadotropin derived from the urine of postmenopausal women. Neither list specifies provider location, although it is clear that both products rely on human female urine as an active ingredient. The price for three vials of Pregnyl (in the online market) is US$36,[10] and similarly US$36 for one vial of Menopur.[11]

that it was predominantly the donations of postmenopausal Roman Catholic nuns that contributed to the company's development of fertility hormones. As noted in a 2016 news article in reference to this history, "The Vatican soon began delivering nun urine by the truckload, with 10 Sisters providing enough pee for one treatment every 10 days" (Hillsman 2016). However, difficulties meeting the demand for urine led Serono to artificially create FSH—today sold as Gonal-F—effectively making the need for postmenopausal women's urine obsolete, in the case of Serono at least.

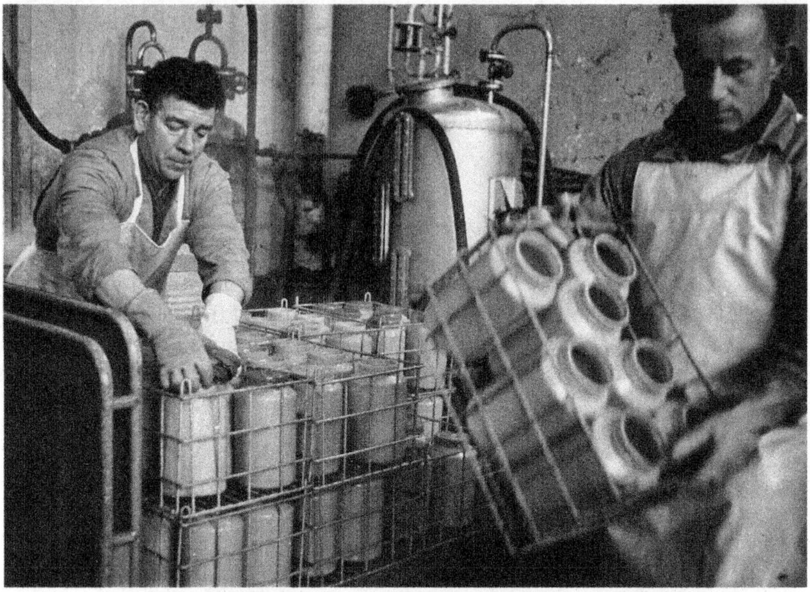

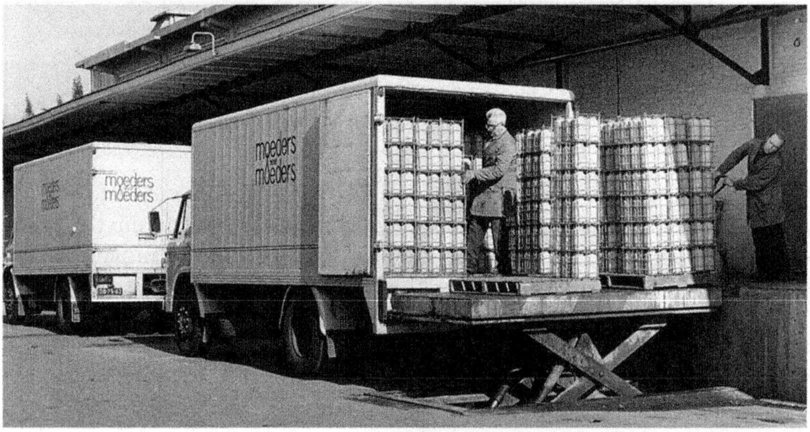

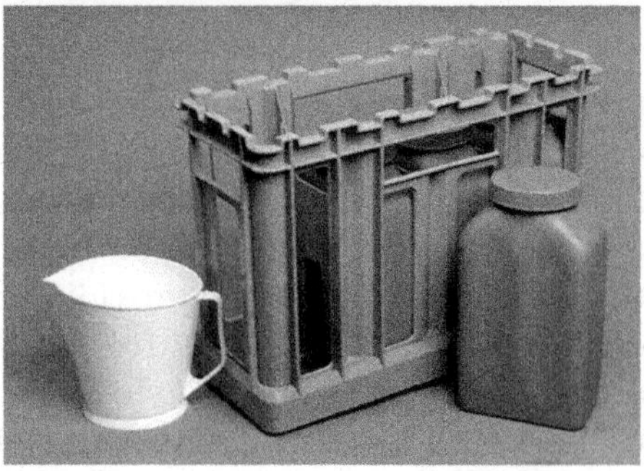

FIGURES 2.3, 2.4, and 2.5. The work involved in early urine collection and production is shown in figures 2.3 and 2.4. Figure 2.5 shows the white pitcher used by the provider in her urine collection (located to the left of the photo). The urine provider pours the collected urine into one of the plastic containers and puts the containers outside (or in a prearranged area) once a week for pickup. All photos courtesy of Moeders voor Moeders.

With a history dating back to 1931, MvM is the oldest remaining urine-collection site. Affiliated with Aspen Oss, MvM is owned by Aspen Pharma, a global pharmaceutical company with headquarters in South Africa. Aspen Pharma has twenty-six pharmaceutical manufacturing facilities spread throughout eighteen locations.[12] MvM facilitates the direct contact with urine providers and covers the entire Netherlands. Through the work of five field managers (all female) and 113 female information providers, MvM introduces and guides pregnant women through the urine-providing process. Urine providing consists of a set of routinized practices in which women collect their urine in a pitcher provided by MvM, pour the collected urine into the bottles provided by the organization (typically eight bottles a week), and then place the bottles outside the front door for the driver to pick up (unless other arrangements have been made). The chauffeur replaces the filled bottles with new ones and the urine is then brought to the factory, first in Boxtel and later in Oss. When collected, the urine is sent from the individual site of collection to the factory in Boxtel, where eight male employees run the first line of purification. Following the initial round, the urine is then sent to Oss for further processing where it is turned into powder, which is then sold to the pharmaceutical company MSD, located next to Aspen Oss, as the necessary active ingredient in Pregnyl. Having briefly outlined the historical and reproductive medical context along with the procedures undertaken for urine donations to take place, I now address the ways that urine enters a global assemblage of waste, care, and value.

Liquid Gifts: Assemblages of Care, Containers, and Gold

> You probably don't think about it when you pee, but your urine contains valuable substances.[13]

> Every drop counts! Due to the need for a lot of urine, every participation is vital.[14]

While urine in many ways exemplifies (reproductive) waste, it is reframed discursively and also materially as a form of gifting, even as a form of love and care, when situated in a donation practice. In what follows, I turn to three analytical incisions in which urine is repositioned as love and care; as waste, as medicine, and as a form of reproductive management; and finally, as a smelly, yet eco-friendly, secret substance. I end the chapter by discussing the ways in which urine providing comes together in this affective, discursive, and technological assemblage to form three imagined, reproductive bodies—the pharmaceutical body, the philanthropic body, and the disciplined, yet porous, reproductive body—prior to turning to a brief discussion of the ways in which urine providing, in the empirical material, intersects with other bodily fluids such as blood and breast milk. Notably, urine, like blood, entangles not only with notions of gifting and sister solidarity but also with nationalized understandings of Dutch solidarity. Yet because the urine is a female-shared fluid, similar to breast milk, I draw on feminist research on the cultural meanings of breast milk to show the ways that the meaning of urine in this material is fluid as well.

Analytical Incision 1: Urine as Enactments of Maternal Care and Sisterly Love

Throughout the Moeders voor Moeders site, providing other women with your urine is spoken of as being an act of maternal care. On the company website, as well as in the provider accounts, urine providing is constructed as a means of creating bonds between similar (but anonymous) predominantly white women, who are united in their desire for maternity yet separated by their ability to become pregnant. Boyer's concept of "caring at a distance" (Boyer 2009: 6), used in the analysis of breast milk donation, is relevant here as well. Boyer notes that breast milk creates care relationships between distant strangers, theorized in her work as the "geography of care" in the creation of a politics of mobile biosubstances (Boyer 2009: 10). Conradson (2003) similarly points to care relationships and notes that care consists of both a set of relationships and also spaces and practices of care that frequently depend disproportionally upon women's care work. While the breast pump, in the case of breast milk donation, turns milk into a mobile biosubstance, in the case of urine providing, the combination of the white pitcher (to pick up urine) and generic blue bottles (to save urine) enables urine mobility. Meanwhile, the giving of urine is constructed, more like blood donation (Waldby and Mitchell 2006), as a patriotic means to remedy the perceived trauma associated with female infertility.

On the Moeders voor Moeders website, the provider's identity as a caring individual takes center stage. In the presentational and recruitment video,[15] the text "every change begins with you" is combined with the lyrics and music of Katie Melua's "Thank You Stars." In this combination, Moeders voor Moeders composes a love story in which similarly minded and predominantly white women unite in their dreams and desire for sister-solidarity, motherhood, and the making of a healthy baby. *Every change begins with you,* we are told at the beginning of this promotional video. The video consists of a series of still images that are tied together through Katie Melua's compelling lyrics and music. The still image of the bathroom sign, present early in the video, reminds us what this is about, but it is quickly replaced with a child who holds a huge rock in its place, an image of strength and determination, as well as individual white women who are either positioned in a meditative lotus position or getting ready to enter a running race (seemingly each with herself—perhaps a race against her biological clock?). Other still images include another white woman who runs through a cornfield on a summer day, one who swims under water, another who walks alone on a pier, and one who dances on a white/golden sand beach dressed in an airy white outfit. In each of these activities, the women are portrayed as alone yet also determined and self-reflective, mirroring the responsible reproductive citizen who pursues her life goals and dreams. During this, the text sets the tone of self-discovery (*"discover yourself"*), independence (*"and if it is necessary, you will do it alone"*), and freedom. The still images represent physically strong, able-bodied, balanced, confident, young, white individual women, who are determined to make a difference. The choice to include a still image of a white horse signifies vitality and fertility, while the actual reproductive matter—urine—or the actual providers—pregnant women who squat, collect, and place urine outside their door—including the containers used for collection and the drivers who pick them up, are not present at any point. Instead, the rhetoric of "difficulty," "discovery," and "pushing yourself" and the image of individualized solitude, reflection, care, and gratitude entangle with an assemblage of white, beautiful, young, energetic, able, European female bodies with differently colored hair.[16] These are images that get replaced later in the video with a woman looking into a small opening, another one who appears happily pregnant, and a 2D black-and-white ultrasound image of a fetus.

Toward the end, the video features objects of desire, including a seemingly healthy, young blonde girl, small pink baby shoes resting on a protruding belly, and a newborn baby. The urine, the squatting provider, the containers, the drivers, the Aspen Oss factory workers, the fertility product, and the needles used in conjunction with Pregnyl to stimulate follicles are all completely absent. With the chorus *"So thank you stars,"* the video ends with two pregnant bellies facing off against each other, thereby framing urine providing within a recognizable, rhetorical frame of neoliberal gifting, exemplified in individual, attractive, white, able-bodied, young women who demonstrate their strength, integrity, and fertility by granting others the chance of pregnancy. These are the women who come to display a form of nationalized sister solidarity—in large part because of the choice to use Dutch subtitles throughout the video and visually portraying a predominantly white visual of what could be Western European women. In this process of care, the work involved in urine providing is absent, while the care that promises urine providers a combination of mental and physical insights in the sharing of urine as a global fluid is present. Here, urine turns into love and care. The prospective provider is positioned as a generous, maternal body from which urine providing is retold as an inherent and innate care toward self and others.

This narrative is echoed in the provider accounts as well. Here, urine collection comes across as a naturalized caring practice, and, when mixed with personal stories about infertility, the work that goes into collecting, pouring, and placing the urine bottles outside the door is made to appear minimal, even trivial: "The day I found out that I was pregnant, I immediately signed up with Moeders voor Moeders. Finally, I could give back and hopefully help other couples experience this happiness,"[17] one provider recounts on the organization's website. In these narratives, not only urine but also pregnancy and maternity are presented as bliss: "I happily give all my pee in the hope that somewhere there is a woman who can then step into this beautiful, special world and leave the darkness behind."[18] Whereas urine becomes the fluid that potentially supports the mobility from infertility to fertility, the MvM recruitment material along with the provider accounts also work by constituting a very particular maternal body: a giving, healthy body oriented to others. As echoed by Stearns (1999) in her analysis of breastfeeding in the United States, it is a body that is disciplined and marked by discretion, asexuality, and most notably also self-sacrifice within the context of urine providing.

In the provider narratives available on the Moeders voor Moeders website, urine is constructed as a naturally shared fluid, moving from the private realm of the individual woman's home to outside her door, into a van, and then into the public realm of the factory and the transnational pharmaceutical industry. As echoed in one account, "You can never be too busy to help other people. All you have to do is to pee—which you have to do anyhow."[19] And as reiterated in another, "I have now been busy collecting urine for one week and it does not bother me at all. Whether I have to pee in the toilet or in a pitcher—I am just happy that I can help in this way."[20] So urine providing is positioned as a sensible circulation of a natural process (something "you have to do anyhow"), reiterated within the context of a collectivized desire for pregnancy and maternity that is frequently attributed to women ("I am happy to help"). Consequently, in these testimonies, urine providers enact good maternal bodies that collectively come together on the website to help other women reach maternity. As noted by Valentine (2005) on blood donation, urine providing becomes an imagined community of equally minded providers. Like blood, urine is in the marketing material as well as in these online accounts, depicted as a "public, circulatable fluid" (Valentine 2005: 116). It is a fluid that importantly does not enact or bear kinship. Instead, it becomes a kinship-making tool in the sense that it unites (white, similar-looking, and similarly aged) women in their naturalized desire for motherhood.

Analytical Incision 2:
Urine as Evidence, Medicine and Reproductive Management

Urine predominantly consists of water (approximately 95 percent). It additionally contains nitrogen and, in the case of pregnant women, the placenta-produced hormone hCG, or HMG in the case of postmenopausal women. Excreted from the kidneys, urine is obviously bodily waste. Frequently thought of as a cleaning mechanism, the kidneys remove toxins from the body, balancing water and sodium levels while also returning some of the substances into the bloodstream. This mechanistic view of the kidneys is echoed on the American Kidney Fund website: "Every day, your kidneys filter about 30 gallons of blood to remove about two quarts (half a gallon) of extra water and waste products. The waste products in your blood come from the food you eat and the use of your muscles. This waste and extra water make up your urine" (American Kidney Fund 2016).[21] In this analytical incision, I will discuss how, through the pregnancy test, in the MvM marketing material, and in clinical accounts, urine comes to be understood as medical evidence, actual medicine, and, when crossing human and animal borders, a form of reproductive management.

Early morning urine is best to use in MvM's home-pregnancy test. Today, Aspen Oss uses pregnant women's urine to produce a take-home pregnancy test that detects hCG.[22] According to the National Institute of Health (NIH),[23] using urine to test for pregnancy dates back to 1350 BCE, when, if she suspected a pregnancy, a woman would urinate on wheat and barley to simultaneously also reveal the sex of the offspring. It was not until the 1970s, however, that urine-based pregnancy tests became widely available. Up until that time, pregnancy testing in the United States was done through a blood test, a hormone withdrawal test (later banned), a pelvic exam, or a urine test performed in the doctor's office (Layne 2009). Upon the development of the take-home pregnancy test, women could detect pregnancies earlier, and most importantly women could do the test at home. While the home-pregnancy test has been scrutinized for reliability and accuracy (Gnoth and Johnson 2014), it has been celebrated as a liberating reproductive technology for women, cited as a "low-tech" woman-friendly product (Layne 2009: 75; Siegel 2014). Applying a critical feminist cultural perspective to the pregnancy test, Layne (2009) notes that the pharmaceutical industry became the main benefactor of the take-home pregnancy test.[24] Similarly, Siegel (2014) notes that upon purchasing the home-pregnancy test, she had in fact begun a technology- and consumption-oriented prenatal care system.

In pursuit of a feminist perspective on low-tech reproductive technologies, Layne (2009) illustrates the workings of a critical, cultural approach. Not only is the home-pregnancy test an integral part of reproductive consumer culture, she says, but the test also constitutes a disembodied understanding of pregnancy. According to Layne, "Home pregnancy tests fragment, isolate, identify and measure a single element of these changes" (Layne 2009: 66). Referring to the multiple bodily and physiological changes that a pregnancy starts, Layne (2009) notes that none of them show up in the test, and consequently she criticizes the home-pregnancy test for promoting an understanding of pregnancy as being (mostly) hormonal. The test reduces pregnancy to a mere chemical matter, she says. It enables faster and earlier knowledge of a potential pregnancy ("find out 8 days after conception")[25] and is sold in bulk ("bought as a package of five"), yet it does little to reduce women's uncertainty, as a positive pregnancy test result still has to be verified in the doctor's office. A good pregnancy test is comparable to what Casper and Clarke ironically call fast and cheap healthcare (Casper and Clarke 1998: 255). Similarly, Layne (2009) challenges the idea that the home-pregnancy test successfully enables women to be the first to know (it may in fact be the supermarket cashier). As a low-tech and frequently overlooked technology (see also Casper and Clarke 1998), the home pregnancy test has nevertheless profoundly altered women's experience with pregnancy, calling for what Layne terms a "systematic feminist technology assessment" (Layne 2009: 76) questioning whether the home-pregnancy test is "the 'right tool' for the job" (Casper and Clarke 1998).

Not only is urine a core ingredient in the making of Pregnyl and pregnancy tests, it also plays a recognizable role in the assessment and recuperation of medical health. In this analytical incision, urine is not exclusively bodily waste or biomedical evidence, but a medical treatment. In the field of reproduction, urine is turned into medicine, assisting in the management of infertility through stimulating follicular growth and through it being turned into the drug Pregnyl. Meanwhile, the Urine Therapy Association, located in Hong Kong, turns each member's urine into a health drink. In this narrative, drinking your own urine assists with everything from improving poor eyesight to even promoting younger-looking skin: "In these 22 years [of urine therapy], I never caught a cold. My eyesight has become clearer and I don't have any age pigment" (Gan 2014). In this analytical incision, urine becomes an alternative medical treatment—a reinvention in which waste is turned into medicine.

In its capacity as medicine, urine crosses not only the border between infertile and fertile human female bodies but human/animal borders as well. When combined with pregnant mare serum, human gonadotropin is used in the development of the drug PG 600, a product managing sow reproduction. In this product, human gonadotropin enables a move to "reproductive management." The use of PG 600 is articulated by Intervet Netherlands as, "Same time, same place. PG 600 will improve the reproductive management of your herd by inducing heat on schedule. Synchronization allows the best use of housing and easier batching of piglets by age. So you can move them all to the same place at the same time. Time after time after time."[26] In the material, the importance of synchronized mobility is further reiterated in the cover photo of five sows of equal size standing (almost evenly) side by side. Here, we learn that urine-as-reproductive management takes the variables out of reproduction ("reproduction is full of variables"), makes reproduction more efficient ("more piglets per sow per year, PG 600 turns the heat on"), and makes more profits. This is not unlike the use of Pregnyl in IVF treatments, in which urine is positioned as enabling medical doctors to time reproduction: "And they can control this timing thanks to this product," says one of the Moeders voor Moeders recruiters on the company's YouTube video, when informing a prospective provider.[27]

The move from reproductive medicine to reproductive management has not been without its own set of problems, however. When news reports in the mid-1980s revealed that the leftover urine collected by Moeders voor Moeders circulated not as medication used in women's infertility treatments but rather as an element in the reproductive management of sows, the organization's very existence was threatened—with it now teasingly referred to as "Mothers for Sows" (Trommelen 2013). Dutch providers threatened to stop supplying the company with their valuable urine (Trommelen 2013). According to Trommelen's news article, the result was that the organization ended its circulation of Dutch urine into the business of reproduction management; however, MvM enacted the very same program in the late 1980s in Brazil.[28] When the company stopped its operations in Brazil in 2008, it was estimated that 6,000 women provided approximately 170,000 liters of urine a month, assisting in the continued development of products like PG 600 (Trommelen 2013). In this context, urine has promissory value and becomes "biological capital" (Rajan 2016), as argued by Gupta and Richters (2008), which is deposited in biotechnology banks and turned into resources from which the pharmaceutical companies can draw.

Analytical Incision 3: Urine as a Stinky and Eco-friendly Secret Flow

During pregnancy, hormonal changes increase the frequency of urination, the volume, and potentially also the smell of it. In fact, increased urination is a sign of pregnancy. Nevertheless, urine is frequently seen as both unclean and stinky. In this analytical incision, I turn to the ways that, in online forums and discussion groups, urine providers frame urine as smelly and also as an eco-friendly and secret flow, at times even shameful.

Urine stinks. It is an in-between fluid, an abject (Kristeva 1982), that defies bodily boundaries. As noted by Kristeva in her theory on abjection, "It is thus not lack of cleanliness or health that causes abjection but what disturbs identity, system, order. What does not respect borders, positions, rules. The in-between, the ambiguous, the composite" (Kristeva 1982: 4). On the matter of stink and abjection, but specifically now related to what goes on in the bathroom, Cavanagh extends Kristeva's theory to pose, "Disgust with urine is often about a perceived encroachment upon the border between inside and outside, private and public, self and other" (Cavanagh 2010: 143). Once on the outside of the body, urine turns into a reproductive waste product and potentially contaminates what it gets in contact with. As argued by Cavanagh, "Body fluids left in and around the white, oval porcelain toilet bowl or urinal are met with disgust because they interfere with our internationalized body maps" (Cavanagh 2010: 146). In the online discussion forums, providers manage the smell of urine through the creation of new routinized practices that uphold a particular understanding of how urine is supposed to move:

> Advice on dealing with the smell: I screw the lid off with an outstretched arm. I place the bottle on the edge of the bathtub. Then, I pour the urine with an outstretched arm and turn my head the other way. Then, I almost cannot smell it.[29]

Here, the provider manages the potential disgust of stink (with an outstretched arm), places the bottle in an appropriate place ("on the edge of the bathtub"), and tries to remove two of her senses ("turn my head the other way"). In this management of smell, urine unfolds in an entanglement of intimacy, hygiene, and senses (vision) against the backdrop of urine as a smelly, (potentially always) unhygienic bodily fluid. Interestingly, the providers frequently mention smell either as a barrier in the decision to join the MvM program or as a surprising, unproblematic aspect of urine providing. Frequently considered a lowered sense (compared to vision and hearing [Pink 2009]), it is also gendered, classed, and raced. As noted in Largey and Watson's sociology of odors, smell entangles with race and ethnicity ("the smell of garlic"), class ("stinky sweat" or "the smell of money"), and gender and sexuality ("she smells like a whore" or "smelling like a rose") (Largey and Watson 1972: 1023, 1025). In this manner, smells can be critically contextualized within a white, gendered, Western moral hierarchy of "pure" and seemingly "attractive" smells: "Odors, whether real or alleged, are often used as a basis for conferring a moral identity upon an individual or a group" (Largey and Watson 1972: 1024). In this manner, stink is implicated in angst about urinary spills (Cavanagh 2010) as well as in the ways that health and cleanliness come together in the production of foul (unattractive) smells. This is also evident in the provider (as well as non-provider) accounts, when stink intermixes with disgust as well as fears of contamination:

> I have also been a part of this. But it is totally crazy. The guy who brought and picked up the bottles did not think that I had peed enough. I filled one bottle a week because I simply threw up each time I had to open a filled bottle. The smell of urine—Yikes![30]

> I am still not participating in Moeders voor Moeders. I just really don't think that it is very hygienic. I simply cannot get used to it. Luckily a lot of other people are ready to give their urine to women just like that! And it is not because I don't support it, it just really isn't me. It is a crazy thing. I am sure it has to do with my fear of contamination.[31]

When understood as stink, urine becomes a troublesome fluid ("the smell of urine—Yikes!"). In these accounts, it is a secretive yet also potentially shameful fluid or flow. Whereas pregnant women can participate in the program as early as their sixth week of pregnancy, providers express concerns related to the privacy of their donation. Participation constitutes a public outing of sorts, in which pregnancy leaves the confines of women's own privacy and enters (now in MvM's characteristic blue bottles) into the public arena. Similar to Stearn's (1999) study of breastfeeding, urine providers may initially hide their donation, valuing discretion and secrecy. Meanwhile, the blue bottles signify participation in the MvM program, leading the organization to respond to the question, "Can I still keep my pregnancy a secret?" with a "Yes, definitely. The contact person can definitely find a solution to where the bottles can be hidden so that your surroundings do not find out whether or not you are pregnant. Arrange that with her. Besides, there is no MvM advertisement on the vehicle that picks up the urine."[32] Secrecy is not always a reality, however. As noted by one provider who chooses to drop the bottles off herself (instead of having them picked up), and in response to the significance of the public arena in making her donation visible to outsiders, "I do not think that the drivers are discreet enough (during my last pregnancy, the whole street knew about it during the seventh week)."[33] And even when contained within the privacy of the home, the procedure for urine providing can prove challenging at best: "My husband does not think it is sexy to listen to, plus every now and again, my daughter runs around with the pitcher in her hand, if she has been in the bathroom, and happily yells: Mommy's piss."[34]

In the provider as well as the MvM marketing material, urine is not only stinky, it also turns into an eco-friendly flow. In this narrative, what has the appearance of a natural waste product enters into an environmentally friendly ecosystem and returns to nature as a fertilizer product. Although not referencing the production of fertilizer, one provider underscores urine providing as an eco-friendly flow when she notes that there is a double advantage to urine providing: It helps some women, while it also saves water:

> Of course you are thinking, "Yikes—to have to collect your urine daily in a pitcher." But what is really troublesome about it? It saves a lot of water and you make a lot of other women (and men) happy by doing it. And of course, every now and again you think, "I really do not feel like collecting it right now." But the feeling of having made a difference gets you going. If every now and again I am not able to collect my urine, then I can hear myself whisper "sorry" in the toilet, because it feels like a wasted opportunity.[35]

Similarly, MvM undertakes a green approach in its decision to transport leftover urine once a week to another Dutch company, GMB Watertechnologie te Tiel, SaNiPhos, and thereby contributes to the production of fertilizer, thus turning a profitable pharmaceutical ingredient into an "environmentally-friendly project."[36] In SaNiPhos's own marketing material, a photo of two men using public urinals is replaced with a close-up of a young woman smiling (seemingly at a music festival) with the text, "How green are your events?" The visual presentation of SaNiPhos and the morally superior production of "green" fertilizer are reinforced through photos of a female medical doctor, fresh-looking fruits and vegetables, and two children (a girl and a boy), seemingly healthy and outdoors, with the girl eating an apple.[37] MvM's contribution appears in the SaNiPhos marketing material as well. A photo of a white pregnant woman, who is resting on a couch dressed in all-white clothes, appears next to a presentation of the MvM program. The pregnant woman smiles, and her very protruding, naked pregnant belly signals a comfortable yet renewed return to nature. In this manner, urine is recast as an eco-friendly flow—including the leftover urine. It is an admirable effort to improve women's chances of an "own" pregnancy. In MvM's collaboration with this environmentally friendly Dutch corporation, the urine of the male festival participants, when mixed with pregnant women's leftover urine, is made to incorporate and re-enchant nature (Smith 1998) in the production of new eco-friendly substances and healthy foods (such as the delicious-looking fruits and vegetables).

Imagined Provider Bodies

At first glance, urine providers are fairly anonymous female bodies. Women undergoing IVF might be surprised to know that pregnant women's urine constitutes the main active ingredient in the drug

Pregnyl. But at the same time, as previously noted, urine does not have the power to create kin, unlike DNA or even blood. Pande challenges the notion of kin through genes when, in her analysis of surrogacy in India, she argues that blood (the shared substance) and sweat (pregnancy work) make kinship: "Kinship established by 'shared substance' allows for one way of reconceptualizing relationships as process. Forms of relatedness that are made viable by 'kin work' are other instances of everyday forms of relatedness" (Pande 2009: 387). This can hardly be said of urine. In this section, I discuss the ways that, in the recruitment material, in the online accounts, as well as in and through affects and routinized practices, urine providers appear as specifically normative bodies—altruistic, disciplined, and maternal—which are conceptualized in the remaining part of this chapter as pharmaceutical, philanthropic, and disciplined yet porous bodies.

The Pharmaceutical Body

The use of pregnant women's urine in the creation of Pregnyl produces an understanding of the female body as a pharmaceutical one. Martin's (2006) delineation of the pharmaceutical person is appropriate. The pharmaceutical person is a self-enhancing person who consumes pills not only to become a better person but in fact also to become the very person he or she really is—just without the particular disorder that the medication is supposed to manage. This is also how Martin frames the "pill person" or the pharmaceutical person (Martin 2006: 275). According to Martin (2006), the "pill person" must also be understood as a product of the branding that goes into the pharmaceutical industry. She quotes a CEO of a small advertising agency, noting that the successful pharmaceutical brand effectively transforms the pill into a person: "We want to get an idea of, if this drug was a person, what kind of person would it be? What would they look like, what do they feel like?" (Martin 2006: 275). In this subsection I discuss the pharmaceutical body not only in regard to the urine provider's body (as a site of pharmaceutical resource and production) but also in regard to the receiver's body (the pill person or body as a site in need of reproductive assistance). Meanwhile, urine providers, like breast milk providers, share their vitality. This is in contrast to "banking" or "investing" it (such as in the case of egg freezers or placenta stem cell banking), where the depositor's reproductive or health future is at stake (Boyer 2009).

Upon agreeing to participate in the program, the urine provider is visited by one of the 113 female MvM information providers. In the film clip of an MvM information provider, we follow Irma's arrival into Elise's home. We see Elise's positive pregnancy test (two strips indicating a positive pregnancy) while the camera centers on Elise's clean, modern, and attractive Dutch home. The two women sit across from each other in the dining room. In the background, a balcony and what appears to be a new white kitchen are visible, while the camera quickly displays the wedding ring on Elise's hand. The video ends with Elise receiving a small gift (a white baby towel in a small MvM bag). In this meeting, Irma explains the purpose of MvM to Elise and emphasizes hCG's ability to "time" ovulation, which is necessary in the treatment of infertile couples. In this information meeting, Irma presents the hCG hormone as shared and makes reference to the hormone's ability to, in other women, develop viable oocytes ("What this is really about is hCG, the pregnancy hormone. This hormone has the ability, aside from what it does to you"). It turns into a sort of generic assistance ("helping other couples gain access to this product") and a reproductive management tool ("It is really important, during a fertility treatment, that you can 'time' ovulation"):

> "Okay Elise. What this is really about is hCG, the pregnancy hormone." [*Irma looks directly at Elise, smiles, and proceeds to show her a graph illustrating the availability of hCG in Elise's urine during the first part of pregnancy. The graph vividly shows the presence of hCG during the ten-week period of pregnancy*] "This hormone has the ability, aside from what it does to you. It was at some point found out that it has a positive effect on ovulation. This effect can be used during IVF but also during IUI [intrauterine insemination]. It has to do with insemination. It is really important, during a fertility treatment, that you can 'time' ovulation. And they can control this timing thanks to this product. And because you are participating, you are helping other couples gain access to this product. I assume that this was also your intent and the reason for participating in the program?"[38]

In the above account, Elise's body turns into a pharmaceutical production body. While no mention is made of MvM's or Aspen Oss's economic incentives, the historical contextualization of hCG is only briefly highlighted ("It was at some point found out that it has a positive effect on ovulation"). Void of the medical and economic detail, Elise's pharmaceutical body is positioned as valuable, as well as readily shared with others ("other women"), reiterating also, through the visual representation of Elise's wedding ring, a particular understanding of the normative heterosexual recipient couple.

Whereas providers can be understood as pharmaceutical producers, the pharmaceutical body takes center stage in the Pregnyl advertisements aimed at consumers. Here, urine turns into a valuable pharmaceutical *product*, transforming the provider's pregnant body into a resource producing affects of hope and desire on behalf of infertile couples, effectively positioning pregnancy and childbearing as not only desirable but natural. In the ad for Pregnyl 5000IU, the infertile woman is visually portrayed as a damaged body, which, combined with a strained heterosexual relationship (the man sits with crossed arms, signaling a closed, non-approachable body, even fading into the background), exudes affects of desperation and loss.[39] The white female reproductive body is here portrayed as an affective but also mechanistic body: she is clearly distraught, and the ad suggests to take Pregnyl 5000IU in order to solve infertility issues. In this visual representation, the pharmaceutical body emerges as a mechanistic one, or as noted by Martin, "When the female body is seen as a mechanical production device, irregularity is understood as pathology, and efforts are made to restore regularity" (Martin 1998: 73). Meanwhile, in the ad, this Pregnyl ("Buy Effective hcg Pregnyl") product promises to solve infertility—now reframed as a disorder—along with the heterosexual romantic relationship, portrayed visually as strained.

The notion of the pharmaceutical body is similarly present in the commercials advocating the so-called hCG diet. While MvM takes a strong stance against the use of hCG as a weight-loss tool, the weight-loss industry itself embraces the use of hCG. For example, in the commercials for what is framed as the fast hCG diet, women are promised to lose weight quickly.[40] A healthy-looking white female with long brown hair, dressed in tight-fitting clothes, stands with a bowl of fruit, enticing the viewer to go on the hCG diet, which consists, as visually documented in the ad, of a needle and various medications. Similarly, yet this time in a televised commercial, obesity is solved through a low-dose hCG diet, helping to balance metabolism and to get rid of "unattractive fat" through what is framed as "an all-natural product." In the commercial, hCG is narrated as a "clinical approach to the treatment of obesity," without mentioning the use of pregnant women's urine. It is positioned as *easy*, and weight loss is rhetorically framed as "essentially guaranteed." While obesity in this television commercial is positioned as a "bodily disorder," hCG is seen to combat "abnormal fat," which is defined as the fat that is "unattractive and never seems to go away," portrayed by a picture of a nude male upper body with a huge stomach and sagging breasts. Within the context of the weight-loss industry, hCG becomes a wonder drug ("It will solve all of your problems"). So the obese body is constructed as a bodily disorder, understood to be imbalanced and out of control due to the presence of this excessive amount of "abnormal fat."[41] The circulation of urine into the weight-loss industry is illustrative of the ways that urine and hCG move from one pharmaceutical context to another, contributing to an understanding of the reproductive body as a pharmaceutical one.

The Philanthropic Body

In the marketing material, recruitment videos and provider accounts available on the MvM website, and interviews with MvM, urine providers are constructed as philanthropic female bodies, or as noted by one woman, "You make the world a better place."[42] In these narratives, the discomfort of pregnancy is replaced with the pride and accomplishment associated with providing other women with a chance of motherhood. The work that goes into urine providing is made to appear manageable—employing gendered somatic work ("I do it with a smile")—as well as necessary ("perhaps you who are reading this need me so badly"). Along with the maternal and philanthropic body, women's reproductive bodies are understood as a sort of ecosystem. As noted by Franklin et al. (2000), body environmentalism has produced a shift from the mechanistic view of the body to one in which the body is an ecosystem. In this discourse, urine not only becomes a carrier of meaning (a symptom, a treatment, and potentiality—hCG), it also becomes a good cause: "But you do help a lot of women doing it and so I am willingly squatting for the cause."[43] As noted by Franklin et al., this shift in understanding of the body as an ecosystem involves new imperatives that I will return to in the next section, including "the responsibility to maintain balance, the need to keep oneself informed, the duty to calculate risks" (Franklin et al. 2000: 41).

> I really do advise all pregnant women to participate! I was so lucky that I have not had any nausea and could therefore withstand the smell from the blue bottles. ☺ But even if you have nausea, it really makes you feel great to be able to do this![44]
>
> Of course, I have also started the "peeing in the pot" and I do it with a smile. Knowing that someone else—perhaps you who are reading this—needs me so badly.[45]

However, from the perspective of feminist scholars, reproductive philanthropy must be understood critically (Dickenson 2009; Sharp

2000; Scheper-Hughes 2015; Strathern 1988). The philanthropic reproductive body draws heavily on gendered understandings of the legitimate maternal body (gift-giving and self-sacrificial). Boyer (2009) illustrates this in her research on breast milk donations, in which women are seen to share their substances willingly and happily. Moreover, the fact that some of these bodily exchanges are undertaken within the home (urine as well as breast milk) has the effect of granting them the appearance of being natural and even innate—disguising the work that goes into them. Addressing the issue of breast milk donations, Boyer's notion of "caring at a distance" is pertinent, enabling "care relationships between distant strangers" and simultaneously turning women's reproductive bodies into "socio-technical assemblages" of care fluids (Boyer 2009: 6, 8). I will return to the gift-giving narrative inherent in the construction of the philanthropic and eco-friendly body in this book's conclusion, but for now I will note that philanthropy has the effect of making the circulation of urine appear natural and rightful. Meanwhile, the entanglements between reproductive fluids and economic and industrial interests are strikingly absent. As noted by Boyer, this involves the fact that "corporate third parties are increasingly profiting from biosubstances harvested for free" (Boyer 2009: 14). In the case of MvM, the philanthropic body, along with the decision to use leftover urine in the production of fertilizer, establishes an understanding of MvM as not only involving philanthropic female bodies but also being a rightful and eco-friendly organization itself.

The Disciplined yet Porous Female Body

How do women discipline their bodies and reproductive fluids to participate in the Moeders voor Moeders program? And what does this act of disciplining do to the understanding of women's reproductive bodies? As noted by Sawicki, reproductive technologies can readily be seen as discipline technologies that render "women's bodies more mobilizable in the service of changing utilities of dominant agencies. Their aim is less to eliminate the need for women than to make their bodies even more useful. They enhance the utility of women's bodies for multiple shifting needs" (Sawicki 1999: 193). In the case of urine providing, routinized practices such as the home visit, a pitcher, and blue bottles produce the idea of a disciplined and manageable, clean flow. Providers are informed that "every drop counts," while routinized practices simultaneously enable easy participation: women are given eight bottles to fill ("a new clean bottle each day"), while bottles are picked up (depending on the location) after work hours ("in your case, Amsterdam is in the evenings")[46]:

Elise: Is it only morning urine that you collect?

Irma: No. It can be urine all throughout the day. I have two pitchers for you, and as a matter of fact, you need to collect as much urine as possible. All throughout the day really. Yes literally, every little drop counts. You collect it in these [bottles], and I have brought a box with me as well. And a number of bottles and in each of these bottles is a little bit of conservation media that makes sure the urine stays fresh without you having to have it refrigerated. So you can also keep these bottles in the shed.

Elise: And how many bottles do I get?

Irma: You get two boxes from us with eight bottles in total. It means that you start with a new clean bottle each day.

Elise: And when are the bottles picked up?

Irma: The bottles are picked up once a week at a prearranged time. And in your case, Amsterdam is in the evenings. The rest of the Netherlands, it is during the day. Here is everything that I have already told you, repeated once more [*gives Elise a brochure*]. And then I brought you a nice gift.

Elise: How nice. Thanks so much.

Thus, while collection and especially pouring the urine into the bottles are considered troublesome in several accounts, these providers are nevertheless viewed as flexible enough to engage in this type of reproductive work. On the topic of flexibility, Longhurst notes that "women's bodies are often considered to be 'naturally' more pliable, supple, bendable, limber, yielding, adaptable and compliant—in short, more flexible than men's" (Longhurst 2004: 119). Moreover, because the actual collection and pouring is undertaken in the privacy of the bathroom, urine providing is undertaken in a very particular disciplinary space: "There is something about toilets/bathrooms and the (excremental) bodies that they house that constructs them as an 'unspeakable space'—a close(t) space—in geographical discourse. Toilets/bathrooms tend to be considered too material, too squeamish, too uncomfortable, too unacceptable (or just plain too banal) to discuss" (Longhurst 2004: 129). Considering also the observation that the bathroom is frequently viewed as an "abject zone" (Kristeva 1982), where what is inside the body makes its way out and escapes bodily boundaries, urine providers discipline their flow in this zone through "clean" pickup and pouring into the blue (clean and neutral) MvM bottles.

Following the work of Rose (2007) and Martin (1998), this type of self-management can aptly be understood as the reenactment of a post-Fordist, ethical, and responsible reproductive citizenship project. To Rose (2007), responsibility relates to the management of future (reproductive) health. Yet reproductive management can also be seen as the self-discipline and responsibility that, in this case, women enact when they correctly facilitate what Martin calls the "flow of information" (Martin 2009: 75). In the case of Elise above, she manages her urine providing through appropriate collection and drop off while maintaining responsible reproductive citizenship through her decision to participate in the MvM program. In this manner, the everyday pregnant body is put into new use through disciplinary and regulatory routinized practices.

From Waste to Liquid Gold

In this chapter I have combined a more historical account of the development of hCG with urine providers' stories, the technical apparatus used to fill the bottles and transport urine (pitcher and bottles), marketing material, and films to discuss the ways that pregnant women's urine (e)merges as a global fluid in this assemblage. In these accounts urine is neither a part of the self nor belonging to someone else. It is reproductive waste. However, as renewed valuable waste, urine readily enters into an emergent pharmaceutical and reproductive management industry. Pregnant women's urine is constructed as the "right" active ingredient in the making of the fertility hormone Pregnyl and in the decision to rhetorically and visually unite Dutch pregnant women in a sort of sister solidarity. Similar to Casper and Clarke, I note that "'rightness' and 'wrongness' are socially constructed, relative, partial, situated and contingent" (Casper and Clarke 1998: 257). I have demonstrated throughout this chapter how urine—an inexpensive resource to MvM—turns into an assemblage of sister solidarity and liquid gold through standardized procedures, provider discipline, urine pickup arrangements, factory processing facilities, and a nationalized discourse of altruism.

Notes

1. Merck Sharp & Dohme is a company based in New Jersey, USA, which acquired Organon in 2007. Up until then, Organon was a pharmaceutical ingredient producer, headquartered in Oss. Organon can be traced back to 1923, when Dr. Saal van Zwanenberg produced the first insulin product in Oss.

2. The Danish International Review Board, affiliated with the University of Southern Denmark, exempts interview studies from IRB application. However, in its attempts at providing all participants with openness and integrity, the project adhered to the European Science Foundation (ESF) guidelines: http://ec.europa.eu/research/participants/data/ref/h2020/other/hi/h2020-ethics_code-of-conduct_en.pdf (retrieved January 2016). This case study relies more heavily on internet based research, however. Consequently, I have especially paid attention to the considerations outlined by the Association of Internet Researchers emphasizing a contextual understanding of "harm," "risk" and the vulnerability of the author/informant. More information can be found at A. Markham and E. Buchanan, "Ethical Decision-Making and Internet Research: Recommendations from the AoIR Ethics Working Committee (Version 2.0)," AOIR: Association of Internet Researchers, December 2012, https://aoir.org/reports/ethics2.pdf (retrieved February 2016).
3. Rich Earth Institute, located in Vermont, advocates for urine-diverting toilets that keep urine separate from the wastewater stream and, thus, enables collected urine to be used as a resource instead. More can be read under the category "Urine Diversion," available at http://richearthinstitute.org/our-work/urine-diversion/ (retrieved January 2016).
4. This estimate is based on the calculations carried out by Rich Earth Institute: "Farming," http://richearthinstitute.org/rethinking-urine/farming/ (retrieved April 2016).
5. Similar to Rich Earth Institute, attempts at rethinking the use of urine is undertaken in the Netherlands. More about these attempts can be read at: http://www.parool.nl/parool/nl/1024/GROEN/article/detail/3536666/2013/10/31/Plassen-op-het-Beursplein-voor-een-groener-Amsterdam.dhtml (retrieved January 2016).
6. The term "liquid gold" is used by the Rich Earth Institute to entice the interest of potential new providers: Rich Earth Institute, "Donate Urine," http://richearthinstitute.org/get-involved/donate-urine/ (retrieved April 2016).
7. The project involved two visits to MvM located in Oss in the Netherlands as well as an accumulation of an online archive of media texts either produced by MvM or written about MvM during the time period of 2010 to 2016. The online archive included the MvM website, YouTube promotional videos, as well as pregnancy internet sites in which Moeders voor Moeders was mentioned. To ensure that all relevant material was included, the online archive was created with the assistance of a Dutch-speaking research assistant. All relevant material was then translated into Danish by the research assistant.
8. Aspen Oss can be traced back to 1923 and the Organon corporation. Organon's founder was Saal van Zwanenberg, owner of a slaughterhouse, who began his work extracting animal bodily parts (what were otherwise frequently nonconsumable objects) and turning them into

active ingredients in what is now known as the pharmaceutical industry. More information about Organon and Aspen Oss can be found on the company website: http://www.aspenoss.com (retrieved October 2016).

9. According to an interview with MvM, September 2016.
10. This price is taken from the online store OnlineDrugPills: http://www.onlinedrugpills.net/buy-pregnyl-5000iu-10000iu-hcg-online.html (retrieved October 2017). Prices vary depending on the recipient's location and whether she is covered by (state) health insurance.
11. The price for one vial of Menopur. The price is taken from the IVFMeds website: http://www.ivfmeds.com/MENOPUR/ (retrieved October 2017). Prices vary depending on the recipient's location and whether she is covered by (state) health insurance.
12. Aspen Pharma is a global pharmaceutical company: http://www.aspenpharma.com/group-overview-2/ (retrieved September 2016).
13. This is according to the Moeders voor Moeders site: https://www.moedersvoormoeders.nl/over-ons/belangrijk-om-te-weten/110/samenwerkingsaniphos.html (retrieved June 2016).
14. This is according to the Moeders voor Moeders site: https://www.moedersvoormoeders.nl/contact/veelgestelde-vragen/134/deelname.html (retrieved September 2016).
15. This is according to the Moeders voor Moeders site: https://www.moedersvoormoeders.nl/over-ons/34/wie-is-moeders-voor-moeders.html (retrieved April 2016).
16. This is according to the Moeders voor Moeders site: https://www.moedersvoormoeders.nl/over-ons/34/wie-is-moeders-voor-moeders.html (retrieved April 2016).
17. This is according to the Moeders voor Moeders site: https://www.moedersvoormoeders.nl/ervaringsverhalen/ervaringsverhalen/1347/freena.html (retrieved June 2016).
18. This is according to the Moeders voor Moeders site: https://moedersvoormoeders.nl/ervaringsverhalen/ervaringsverhalen/1190/eltje.html (retrieved June 2016).
19. The video can be accessed through YouTube: https:www.youtube.com/watch?v=LUuWtakGclk (retrieved June 2016).
20. This is according to the Moeders voor Moeders site: https:www.moedersvoormoeders.nl/ervaringsverhalen/ervaringsverhalen/1351/daisy.html (retrieved June 2016).
21. American Kidney Fund, "About Your Kidneys: What Do My Kidneys Do?," http://www.kidneyfund.org/kidney-disease/about-your-kidneys.html#what_do_my_kidneys_do (retrieved October 2016).
22. While the prices of pregnancy tests vary, in the United States they usually run between US$8 and US$10, and in Denmark they cost approximately US$8 when purchased in one of the local pharmacies.
23. The history of pregnancy testing is aptly described by the National Institute of Health. https://history.nih.gov/exhibits/thinblueline/timeline.html (retrieved October 2016).

24. According to Layne, the sale of home pregnancy tests in the United States accounted for $206 million in sales in 1997 (Layne 2009: 70).
25. An example of the marketing of pregnancy tests can be found at the Med24 website: https://www.med24.dk/hjemmetest/graviditetstest/tidlig-graviditetstest-2-stk-/product_info.php/cPath/44_45/products_id/20681?gclid=Cj0KEQjw4rbABRD_gfPA2-uQqroBEiQA58MNdLsnSoT_tC8y6fQtX7w_MLME4IQOIkee4YaAgQp7FcEaAhVA8P8HAQ (retrieved October 2016).
26. This is according to the Intervet marketing material found at The Pig Site: http://www.thepigsite.com/focus/contents/PG600%20061797.pdf (retreived September 2016).
27. This is according to the YouTube video available at: https://www.youtube.com/watch?v=-XCotBIm_OI (retrieved June 2016).
28. According to Trommelen (2013), the company did not inform the Brazilian donors that their urine would be used, at least partially, in the development of reproductive medicine to sows.
29. This is according to an online forum at the Forum voor zwangeren website: http://forumvoorzwangervrouwen.nl/moeders-voor-moeders?page=5 (retrieved June 2016).
30. This is according to a pregnancy forum at the Forum voor zwangeren website: http://www.zwangerschapspagina.nl/zwangerschap/518385-kado-mvm-3.html (retrieved June 2016).
31. This is according to an online forum at the Forum voor zwangeren website: http://forumvoorzwangerevrouwen.nl/moeders-voor-moeders?page=2 (retrieved July 2016).
32. This is according to Moeders voor Moeders: https://www.moedersvoormoeders.nl/contact/veelgestelde-vragen/134/deelname.html (retrieved October 2016).
33. This is according to a pregnancy forum at the Zwangerschapspagina web site: http://www.zwangerschapspagina.nl/zwangerschap/518385-kado-mvm-4.html (retrieved June 2016).
34. This is according to a pregnancy forum at the Zwangerschapspagina website: http://forumvoorzwangerevrouwen.nl/moeders-voor-moeders?page=2 (retrieved June 2016).
35. This is according to Moeders voor Moeders: https://www.moedersvoormoeders.nl/ervaringsverhalen/ervarungsverhalen/1151/tamara.html (retrieved June 2016).
36. This is according to Moeders voor Moeders: https://www.moedersvoormoeders.nl/over-ons/belangrijk-om-te-weten/110/samenwerking-saniphos.html (retrieved October 2016).
37. https://www.gmb.eu/images1/gmb/data/SaNiPhos/GMB_Brochure_Saniphos_def.pdf (retrieved October 2016).
38. Moeders voor Moeders recruitment video: https://www.youtube.com/watch?v=-XCotBIm_OI (retrieved June 2016).
39. Penny Saver, "Buy hcg Pregnyl 5000 iu to Detach Infertility Issues," 11 July 2016, https://www.pennysaverusa.com/classifieds/services/

health-services/medical-treatments/other/usa/california/los-angeles/beverly-hills/90210/buy-hcg-pregnyl-5000-iu-to-detach-infertility-issues-222792062.html (retrieved August 2016).
40. Fast Escrow Refills, "Why Ovidac 5000 Iu Injection Is Used during Pregnancy," updated 21 June 2017, https://fastescrowrefill.wordpress.com/2016/03/28/why-ovidac-5000-iu-injection-is-used-during-pregnancy/ (retrieved April 2016).
41. hcgpregnyl, "hcg pregnyl," YouTube, 6 October 2010, https://www.youtube.com/watch?v=JHTTZlhvtck (retrieved October 2016).
42. This is according to a Moeders voor Moeders forum: https://www.moedersvoormoeders.nl/ervaringsverhalen/ervaringsverhalen/1163/melanie.html (retrieved June 2016).
43. This is according to a pregnancy forum at the Zwangerschapspagina website: http://forumvoorzwangerevrouwen.nl/moeders-voor-moeders?page=4 (retrieved June.2016).
44. This is according to a Moeders voor Moeders forum: https://www.moedersvoormoeders.nl/ervaringsverhalen/ervaringsverhalen/1097/sandra.html (retrieved June 2016).
45. This is according to a Moeders voor Moeders forum: https://www.moedersvoormoeders.nl/ervaringsverhalen/ervaringsverhalen/1313/kim.html (retrieved June 2016).
46. Moeders voor Moeders recruitment video: https://www.youtube.com/watch?v=-XCotBIm_OI (retrieved June 2016).

Chapter 3

Oocytes

From Waste to Assets

What's in an egg? Glued to the microscope, I visually examine an egg cell that has been extracted and is now, upon passing what appears to be its first health test, vitrified—frozen for potential later use. The biologist whose microscope I have borrowed guides me in what I see: maturation, viability, and integrity are important health markers, she says. While she has a trained eye, I am struck by how small, yet still visible, the egg cell is. As it is visually distinct and detached from the female body here, it constitutes usable (future) matter. Egg cells come to personify life (Martin 1991). Through the microscope, they reappear as autonomous and independently gendered bodies (Lie 2012). In this chapter, I explore how oocytes come to matter in concrete entanglements and in cultural imaginations. I use feminist cultural analysis to view oocytes as rhetorical practices (Butler 1993), as material-semiotic nodes (Haraway 1997), and as matter and meaning brought together (Mol 2012), yet I first turn to a brief overview of this chapter's assemblage ethnography.

Oocyte Sites

Doing fieldwork in the Spanish fertility clinic starts with wearing the right clothes: white surgical pants, a long white jacket, a green hat (to hide all of my hair), and white shoes. Accompanied by the (pregnant) female medical doctor from Italy, who is scheduled to perform the first embryo implantation procedure of the day, I enter the operating theater of this reputable fertility clinic, located in a posh Barcelona business district. The clinic appeals to an international group of patients.[1] Today is no exception. On the patient list, available in the surgical room, one word describes each patient: "Italian," "German," "British," "French," "Spanish," and "Lesbian." The choice of foregrounding nationality and homosexuality, along with the last name of the medical doctor, makes it clear that language and patient nationality (all but one couple are presumed heterosexual) determine the choice of fertility doctor. In this operating theater, different languages are spoken, yet words of fear, hope, and excitement are unilaterally expressed. Doctors hug some of the recipients and recipients are complemented for having a full bladder, making the ultrasound images more clearly visible to the attending physician. While several of the doctors enthusiastically insist on my seeing the implantation from their vantage point—sitting between the legs of the recipients—I prefer to observe with a bit of physical distance, noting the choreography that goes into implantation (Thompson 2005). In these observations, doctors and patients come and go, while the Spanish nurse and I stay in the room throughout the day, along with all of the equipment.

The assemblage ethnographic material that goes into this chapter includes observations, interviews, and documents in context (ethical debates, legal briefs, clinical marketing material).[2] During my observations in the Barcelona fertility clinic, I was present for initial consultations with international couples and egg-implantation procedures.[3] I have visited and talked with international coordinators at several Spanish clinics located along the Mediterranean coast, with one medical tourist agency in Prague, and with Danish fertility doctors, who are instrumental in making certain reproductive paths accessible to their patients through more or less formalized collaborations with foreign clinics. I have participated in several oocyte-related events, such as a "Take control of your future fertility" seminar, offered by a London-based fertility clinic, and an egg-freezing seminar for new freezers, carried out by a New York City fertility clinic.[4] I have interviewed foreign recipient couples present at the Barcelona clinic, Danish fertility patients who traveled or were planning to travel to Spain or the Czech Republic during 2010–13, and egg freezers in New York City who had chosen to vitrify their oocytes for later use.[5]

Additionally, the empirical material includes interviews with a small group of what I choose to refer to as oocyte *providers,* who had traveled to Barbados to provide other women with their eggs, along with analyses of a more extensive group of provider accounts, written and submitted following provider trips to Global Egg Donors, an intermediary egg-donor agency located in California.[6] And because oocytes gain cultural significance in specific and localized ethical and legal contexts, I include Danish ethical discussions, legal frameworks, and select marketing material.[7] The choice to use the word "provider" rather than "donor," once again, stems from the desire to step outside of the gift/commodity framework that the exchange in reproductive cells so often finds itself in.

This vastly different material comes from five separate geopolitical locations, situated within different legal frameworks and fertility infrastructures: Denmark (Copenhagen), the United States (New York City), the United Kingdom (London), Spain (Alicante and Barcelona), and the Czech Republic (Prague). Whereas Denmark has become a known destination for sperm donation (Adrian and Kroløkke 2018, Spain and the Czech Republic have become established as destinations for egg donation (Kroløkke 2014). Meanwhile, in the United States and also in the United Kingdom, egg freezing is gaining prominence, and, in the United States, egg-provider agencies enable international clients to "hand-pick" the provider of their choice, custom-making fertility treatment in exotic locations such as Barbados (Carroll and Kroløkke 2017; Kroløkke 2016). The work that goes into this chapter covers different localities and different time periods, yet it jointly centers how oocytes gain meaning in concrete rhetorical, material, and affective contexts. It illustrates how values assigned to oocytes transgress biology and reproductive bodies, entangle with reproductive intentions (to give, to sell, to freeze etc.), and come to be understood as emerging out of different geopolitical locations, cultural imaginations, and in concrete clinical practices.

Walking on Eggshells

Analyzing oocytes is a tricky business. Feminist scholars stress how women's reproductive bodies have become desirable, fragmented biological commodities within neo-capitalist reproductive economies (Dickenson 2009; Raymond 1993; Sharp 2000). In this scholarship, oocytes emerge as globalized fluids/commodities, stratifying reproduction along economic and geopolitical forms of privilege. In what follows I situate oocytes as dynamic and fluid entities. I combine ethnographic observations and interview studies with texts and visual images to develop three analytical incisions: one in which oocytes entangle with waste and (uncertain) investments; another in which oocytes are positioned as gifts and commodities; and finally, an analytical incision in which oocytes gain meaning as tiny cells and own (defined as genetically related) babies. Each analytical incision draws upon and materializes a very specific understanding of reproductive cells and reproductive bodies that are not only gendered but also embedded within particular understandings of the raced, nationalized, and sexed reproductive bodies that I later address as imagined reproductive, rightful bodies.

Analytical Incision 1: Eggs as Waste and Investments

Oocytes may become waste (when unused), recyclable material (when used), and investment material (once frozen). The view of oocytes as waste is readily present in the egg providers' written accounts. Tanya, who traveled from the United Kingdom to California to provide an unknown woman with her oocytes, says, "Each month I have a period and literally flush an egg down the toilet." Similarly, Keri positions her non-donated oocytes as literally wasted: "Here I was having a regular cycle every month and it is just going to waste." To Tanya and Keri, egg cells have zero value to them, situating reproductive cells within a production framework in which the (good) productive female body is an active reproductive one.

The view of oocytes as waste is similarly present in the Spanish marketing material, in which providing eggs is constructed as the giving of "excess" tissue (Kroløkke 2014). Hence, oocytes are positioned as insignificant to the person they came from, yet when recycled are made to appear valuable through the infrastructures of the fertility clinic, most notably through visualization and extraction techniques. Lola comments on this when she emphasizes how eggs are only valuable upon being extracted: "My egg had been like a pearl, worthless in the depths of the sea (in me) until taken out for all to behold and make a difference in someone's life and most importantly the heart (a place where all treasures are kept)." Albeit valuable, eggs are potential waste while situated inside the body, yet they gain worth once extracted.

In the provider accounts as well as in the marketing material directed at potential providers, egg cells appear as both waste and plentitude. Tille, who went to Barbados on her provider trip, says, "If you donate a kidney, that's it, it's gone forever, whereas with eggs, I will have more next month. I lose absolutely nothing in this process. In my mind, it's almost an unwanted period, I would normally be throwing away the eggs I do not want." While Tille has agency in the narrative ("I would normally be throwing away"), oocytes become recyclable "unwanted" matter or tissue drawn from a "natural reserve" of eggs, which otherwise would have gone to waste. To Emma, the quest to recycle her reproductive cells gets tied to the fact that she is single: "A single girl, wasting all of her potential eggs every month." While Emma's oocytes are assembled as waste or matter out of place due to her relationship status (Douglas [1966] 1984), oocytes are also readily recycled within the infrastructures of capitalism and the nuclear family, re-naturalized as belonging to a family that has, as Emma says, the "lingering hopes to conceive, to be able to finally have a family."

Not only do oocytes turn into symbolic or literal reproductive waste once they leave the body as menstrual flows, they also become potential waste when left inside the aging reproductive body. Egg freezing or "fertility preservation" promises to save women's eggs against the dangers of becoming wasteful reproductive material (old, genetically damaged, non-reproductive eggs). It has the effect of making freezing a recognizable and even legitimate activity, redirecting our attention away from the business of freezing eggs to something more recognizable, like "preserving the sacred grounds" or "saving the whales," for example. Its promise lies in keeping women's fertility protected from decay (waste), or as Tina, who chose to undergo egg freezing, noted in reference to other women, "So suddenly they're like, 'Oh, my god! No eggs! What are we going to do?'" So preservation gains legitimacy as a sustainable practice that "saves" or "rescues" what has value—here defined as women's ability to have their own genetically related children. Meanwhile, technologies of extraction, freezing, thawing, IVF, repeated visits, and economic exchanges fade into the background. In this rescue narrative, fertility preservation becomes a gender-equalizing technology that enables women (like men) to postpone parenthood.

Just like plentitude is central in the egg providers' accounts of eggs as waste, the notion of scarcity is central to egg recipients and freezers alike. In the case of egg freezing, oocytes are positioned as scarce resources, making freezing a necessary (uncertain) investment. At the age of forty, Maria sees her frozen eggs as "money in the bank," while Lisa positions her decision to freeze as an "insurance policy": "Oh, this is really good, because I don't have to feel that whole biological clock thing. This is a great insurance policy." Not all of the interviewees see vitrified oocytes as solid investments, however. Lea's decision to have a child after two cycles of frozen oocytes and a total of thirty-two frozen eggs is an example of oocytes, albeit a large quantity, turning into uncertain investments: "I'd made lots of eggs, so I had lots of eggs on ice, but I never felt like I was convinced that they were going to work." This concern is reiterated later in the interview when she says, "I think I'd still feel terrified that I had thirty-two eggs on ice somewhere that were useless." To Lea, it is in fact the birth of her son that transforms her vitrified eggs into a good investment: "Now that I have a child, I feel great about my eggs! . . . I really feel like I have covered all of my bases." As investments, eggs entangle with reproductive control, situating women's fertility as exclusively residing in the eggs.

In the promise of eggs on ice and young eggs, the reproductive body becomes plastic—always capable of being in a state of transformation and transition (Landecker 2007). Plasticity is not merely a technological intervention. As argued by Jordan, it is a rhetorical strategy that is "shaped by the ways that the body can be discussed, by whom, and toward what end, as well as the socio-political implications of people seeking to make their bodies conform to an idealized image" (Jordan 2004: 333). In this entanglement, frozen eggs extend plasticity from the reproductive body to the romantic body. Alice notes, "I've dated different people and I just think—I see my friends that are, well, 'I'm getting to a point where I have to have kids, so I have to . . . but I don't, at least, have to, because I have thirty-two-year-old eggs that are better than thirty-eight-year-old eggs.'" Similarly, Rita successfully used oocyte providing in Spain at the age of fifty-one. She reiterates that young eggs enabled her to become pregnant, thus making her reproductive body at the age of fifty-one transformable into a younger, productive body: "The eggs are the problem. Everything else I am good at."

In fact, younger oocytes become an injection of youth and sensuality. Franklin et al. refer to the consumption of the exotic as a way of getting "getting closer to, and incorporating the stranger" (Franklin et al. 2000: 104). Frozen eggs promise to deconstruct reproductive aging, to modify and improve the female reproductive body, while younger (at times foreign) oocytes hold the promise of a healthy child, coupled with a more sensuous body. This is not only the case for younger women or freezers. In the case of fifty-one-year-old Rita, receiving young oocytes and using sperm donation turned what she frames her "nougat" baby into the product of a passionate Latin affair: "I do also say that I am more and more convinced that it was Antonio Banderas . . . The more I look at her, the more convinced I get [laughs]. People do look at me [laughs], and she looks you know like. . . . That thing that I might have known a Spanish man . . . well of course, sure . . . I could have known a Spanish man." Provider oocytes become an intervention in reproduction, such as in the case of Rita, where traveling to Spain is rewritten into an exotic romantic relationship of sorts (Kroløkke 2016, 2014; Adrian and Kroløkke 2018: 10).

When eggs are viewed as investments, freezing gets understood as a technology of optimization. It creates new understandings of frozen egg cells (useable, healthy, optimal) in contrast with fresh matter (aging, dubious and potentially unhealthy, dried-up, ticking time bomb), making the technological interventions involved in extraction, freezing, thawing, fertilizing, and implantation appear necessary and right. Tina notes that she has three embryos and eggs "saved up for a rainy day"; Ruby emphasizes how egg freezing allows her to do things "naturally": "But I kind of feel like having the eggs frozen, like, having them there, although it's not a guarantee, it kind of lets you live your life, and not . . . and do things kind of in the order that you want to do them, and do things naturally. So I didn't have to say, 'Hey!' after dating for three months, 'OK, although we feel like we're going to be together, let's hurry up and have a baby.'"

Egg freezing does more than simply vitrify reproductive cells; it establishes new understandings of fertility ("it's all in the eggs"), reproductive aging ("the aging and reproductive body as plastic"), and social and romantic relations ("no longer driven by a [desperate] desire to reproduce"), which are whitewashed into a white, middle-class woman's reproductive option (Allen 2016) while simultaneously re-naturalizing the desire for a particular, straight temporality (meet the right guy, date him, fall in love, get married, buy a house, have a child) (Carroll & Kroløkke 2017; Puar 2009). Moreover, fertility preservation becomes a way for women to bank and consume reproduction in the name of exercising reproductive choice. In this context, once they are extracted and frozen, eggs become transmitters or messengers of gender equality. This is echoed in the marketing material of one of the latest IVF businesses in New York City. On their website, Eggbanxx displays a white, blond, light-blue-eyed, slender, physically attractive woman who is looking straight at the viewer.[8] Along with the text "Smart women freeze!" Eggbanxx speaks directly to the white, professional, educated woman to "take control" of her fertility.[9] Maria echoes this when discussing her decision to freeze her eggs: "I applaud them [women who freeze] and I think that they should be applauded for taking their fertility into their own hands."

To Rose (2007), medical technologies have a forward dimension, understood as a process of susceptibility and enhancement. This is also the case when it comes to egg freezing and egg providing. Freezing technologies provide tools to intervene in future health prospects. Egg freezers echo this when they work to accumulate the optimal and magical number of twenty oocytes through healthy living and hormone shots. Freezers count their eggs, at times expressing, like Tina, their anxiety: "I was like, oh, gosh, if I don't have that many eggs left, I better take what I have left, and, you know, keep them." This notion of scarcity is also at the very core of fertility travelers' accounts, in which they relate that traveling to Spain or the Czech Republic provides a chance to get good eggs and enhance the prospects of a healthy child. Moreover, the notion of scarcity is present in the Danish clinical material when, for example, the Copenhagen Fertility Center promises Danish women a minimum of ten oocytes and at least two blastocysts from their collaborators in Estonia or Greece.[10]

In this first analytical incision, I have examined how eggs move between the notions of waste and investments. Eggs can be waste (flushed down the toilet), plentiful (recyclable material), in decay (old eggs), in scarcity/shortage (eggs running out of time, the limited number of eggs), and (uncertain) investments (eggs on ice). They entangle with reproductive intent (the intent to provide other women with eggs, to receive, or to freeze) and are deeply embedded within an economy in reproductive services and tissue banking.

Analytical Incision 2: Eggs as Gifts and Commodities

> This is the best, most selfless gift you can ever give an infertile couple. (Tracy)

The commodification of women's reproductive bodies is a contentious issue in feminist scholarship (Dickenson 2009; Raymond 1993; Sharp 2000). This concern is echoed in the Danish Council on Ethics, an independent board that contributes to Danish legal and public debates. Here, ideas on altruism, combined with little, if any, compensation, are positioned as morally preferable and turned into a nation-building story: "The emphasis must be on community-oriented values by supporting altruistic donations, as well as on the importance of the prospective child who has to live with the knowledge of having another biological mother than the social mother" (Danish Council on Ethics 2013: 14). While compensation frequently entangles with monstrosities and immoralities, also associated with sex work, commodification in the case of eggs can raise questions over reproductive quality. Jane, a Danish woman traveling to Spain for egg providing, expresses this concern about compromised quality when she says, "It is also a little dangerous, because how do you secure quality, I'm thinking? If you are paying a lot of money for it, then, a lot of people may exploit it." I return to the moral economy of reproduction in the conclusion to this book, and instead now prioritize the ways that oocytes are given meaning in this gift/commodity framework.

I begin, however, by noting that the very idea of gift giving does something: it mimics the ideal maternal body—a giving, other-oriented body—simultaneously making a sharp distinction between reproductive matter and the world of commerce (Kroløkke 2014). This is notably the case when it comes to egg providers who are expected to construct "feminine" profiles stressing altruism (Almeling 2009). Pollock concurs and points out that the construction of the feminine egg-provider body is embedded within a narrative of altruism: "Altruism, like maternal drive, is a socially desirable feminine quality. It is the explanation that makes the donor's actions acceptable" (Pollock 2003: 255). Similarly, eggs and altruism intertwine in the Spanish clinic. While each potential egg provider has to undergo various health tests and provide the clinic with a genealogical overview of parents' and grandparents' health and occupational status, the psychologist tells me how each provider should preferably be altruistic as well. To her, women who "only want to do it for money" are undesirable and are frequently, she claims, deselected by the clinic. In this manner, egg providing operates as a normative technology, re-naturalizing particular understandings of (good) feminine and, in the Spanish context, altruistic and anonymous providers.

The "giving of eggs" entangles in the clinical discourses and also the provider accounts with emotional rewards. Providing other women with eggs is portrayed as a win-win situation in which the provider, in exchange for her good-quality eggs, tells of receiving great emotional rewards, coupled with what is recounted as the trip of a lifetime. According to Hannah, "The feeling of gratification can't be described." Sue comments, "To give someone such a unique gift is absolutely an amazing opportunity. It's a miracle, a dream come true. After donating, I got this overwhelming feeling of peace. Just knowing that I gave hope to someone in need of their own little miracle, it made me feel special." This sentiment is reiterated in other provider accounts: Anna relates, "The feeling of giving a gift that cannot be bought has fulfilled my soul in a way that can barely be described. It can only be felt." Lola shares, "The donation process made me a better person. It helped me to help other people in the smallest way that I could make a big difference." The emphasis on emotional compensation, not financial rewards, becomes a strategic tool in making it appear natural and legitimate that particular women (younger women) act as gift givers or reproductive assistants (Kroløkke 2014).

Oocytes become more than gifts—they become gift generators. Providers receive gifts from the recipient couple (frequently orchestrated by the agency) as well as the "gift of seeing new places." Marcia, who traveled to Barbados, combines these different gifts when she says, "It is amazing the joy it generates inside when you are able to give a gift so priceless and important. It was not only a wonderful holiday experience but an uplifting journey." Similarly, Nico, who went from Canada to Cyprus, says, "The time it took to do the procedure and donate eggs was so minimal and fully worth it when you get the experience of traveling to such a faraway and cultural place as Cyprus." In these narratives, providers are located in different moments of the reproductive and commodity cycle: they become objects of desire yet also display a privileged type of femininity, when they spend time shopping for jewelry, blankets, household items, etc. (Kroløkke 2016, 2015a). They become tourists, replacing the necessary and dull treatments (hormones, extraction, vaginal ultrasound imaging) with the excitement of shopping, beaches, and city explorations (Kroløkke 2016, 2015a). In this entanglement, eggs are mobile and shared, while frequently resituated within the fertility clinic as just another treatment. Line, who was planning to travel to Spain for treatment, comments, "We are not buying eggs. We are buying treatment."

Egg providing can aptly be viewed as a type of reproductive and somatic work. Providers are encouraged to display professional care and engage in appropriate behaviors related to their reproductive cells. Lori recounts this type of somatic work when she says in her travel essay, "The next morning I prepared for my retrieval procedure. The day of, you are not allowed to use any products. No body wash, deodorant, shampoo, moisturizer. Nothing. It is very important, as any smell can affect the eggs. I left for the clinic, and before long I was dressed in a gown and booties, connected to an IV (the good kind)." In this entanglement, eggs become precious yet also vulnerable gifts, as well as products. Meanwhile, providers optimize the quality of their eggs, but once the eggs are extracted, providers are expected to remain distant from them.

The ways that oocytes entangle with an economy of gifts reinforce the notion that female fertility is "naturally" shared. In the Spanish clinical context, providers are frequently described as innately "giving," exemplified in the clinicians' insistence of the high rates of organ donation in Spain. Ruby and Mike speculate on this when, following their first consultation in the Spanish clinic, they state, "It was interesting, the doctor said that Spain has the highest rate in the world of donors—of organ donors—so it is part of their culture to be giving. So it puts your mind at rest. I suppose it may sound awful, but the further east you go, concerns would creep in as to how these women who are donating—are they purely doing it as a generous thing or is there something more?" Of course, in the face of high compensation rates, the decision to view eggs as gifts glosses over the ways that the economy in eggs is highly stratified, enabling particular women (young, able-bodied, heterosexual, attractive, university students) to become egg providers. And as these examples suggest, the idea of gifting shapes not only how egg providing is understood, recounted, and remembered but also, in this case, the ways that clinical practices are structured and organized (Kroløkke 2014).

Oocytes move from belonging to a particular woman to becoming a gift, and then becoming reproductive cells with particular traits. To Jhally, this fragmentation is characteristic of consumer culture: "In non-market societies there is a unity between people and goods, but in capitalism there is separation between object and producer" (Jhally 1989: 221). Eggs are mobile, yet through the lens of feminist and consumer scholars, they are simultaneously an expression of individuality (Lury 2011). In the clinical marketing material, eggs are white, brown, educated, easily tanned, heterosexual, Danish quality, temperamental, tall, smart, caring, musical, loving mothers, athletic, etc. (Kroløkke 2014). In an attempt to open up a Danish gamete bank, Ole Schou, CEO of Cryos International, argues that Danish women's oocytes are in fact marketable because Scandinavian genes are "sellable," he says (Thomsen 2016). Positioned as always white, in this discourse, Danish women's genes are constructed as recessive, thereby making them sellable to a wide spectrum of clients (similar to Danish sperm) (Thomsen 2016).

Whiteness and nationality come together in the production and marketing of provider eggs. The Spanish fertility clinic assures whiteness and requests their available Brazilian providers to present a racial history of three generations (compared to the two generations requested of the Russian or Spanish providers, for example).

Meanwhile, recipients are asked to fill out a form detailing their own physical traits (hair color, eye color, height, weight, skin color, etc.). In contrast to the Spanish and Danish setting where the clinic does the matching, the allure of Global Egg Donors is that recipients can choose the provider from a long list that includes photos and detailed descriptions.

In fact, on the Global Egg Donor site, recipients are invited to view race and nationality as an aesthetic category. The agency describes recipient choices as follows: "Women are available for egg donation from many ethnic backgrounds. Their genetic roots are from all over the world: UK, Germany, America, Canada, Africa, Denmark, India, Ireland, Portugal, Italy, France, Asia, Russia and Latin America, to name only a few. Choose between white, women of color and black donors. Many of our egg donors are students at the local universities."[11] In the presentation, skin color is "not simply displaced, but replaced and reworked as an act of choice" (Lury 2011: 167). In this case, reproductive choice gets repositioned to consumer choice. Recipients are here invited to select a provider and are even given the opportunity to select one who presumably has the intellectual abilities needed to attend university.

The commodification of reproduction is both globalized and individualized, drawing upon recognizable metaphors of individualism, control, and choice. The fact that eggs, once frozen and fertilized, are mobile speaks to this. The Copenhagen Fertility Center offers to deliver sperm to one of their collaborators in Estonia or Greece. At the Estonian or Greek clinic, an egg cell from one of the three hundred providers (depersonalized on the website, yet framed as "ready" to help the Danish couples) is fertilized and then transported "back" to Copenhagen. Similarly, reproduction is a combination of control and choice, as seen when the Irish fertility clinic Sims IVF grants recipients the exclusive choice of at least two providers: "You can filter the available donors by hair color, eye color and blood group, which may help you narrow your decision. You are allocated a specific time period on the portal and no other couples are permitted to look online at the time that you are choosing your egg donor."[12] On these sites, recipient choice and consumption are individualized, yet through the reinstatement of choice as natural, they are also collectivized.

When oocytes become gifts and commodities, providing other women with oocytes becomes a form of "pan-femininity" (Franklin et al. 2000) in which Northern European women naturally "consume" the fertility of Southern European women (see also Kroløkke

2014). In one of the Spanish clinics, this move is even naturalized and conceptualized as demonstrative of early European settlements, in which Spain gets situated in the narrative as the center of European demographic developments.[13] Even though eggs are most often conceptualized and mediated as gifts, egg providers transgress the gift/commodity framework in several ways, but the clinical and agency marketing material clearly portrays oocytes as biological commodities with particular traits (educated, dark-haired, blue-eyed, young, outgoing, and gift giving). Oocytes exist within the spheres of production (the factory, the reproductive body), finance (the cost/compensation), and affects (hope, desperation, happiness), and once they are separated from the reproductive bodies that they came from, they may transgress national boundaries and cement the inadequacy of the gift/commodity framework.

Analytical Incision 3: Eggs as Tiny Cells and Own Babies

In "Should I Defrost My Freezer Boys?," Ruth Whippman writes about the unintended consequences of successful IVF: two healthy embryos left in a cryopreservation tank in an industrial area of San Ramon, California. In the article, the "frosties" are brought to life, along with Whippman's maternal feelings: "Every time I picture them, I get a visceral jolt of maternal feeling. Sweethearts, you must be so cold in there without your coats. I am their mother"; and later in the text: "I picture the freezer boys like our sons, waiting for us to come and rescue them with the same crumpled, anxious expressions they wear if I am ever five minutes late to pick them up from preschool" (Whipmann 2016). Throughout her story, the embryos are positioned as gendered children: "freezer boys" and "sweethearts" that demand appropriate maternal attention ("you must be cold in there without your coats"). In this subsection, I take a look at the ways that oocytes are imagined as tiny cells (akin to spare parts), but similar to Whippman's "freezer boys," at times also own babies—rescued and cared for by the fertility clinic and in the cryopreservation tanks.

At first glance, oocytes do not equal future babies, unlike embryos. While this is certainly the case in clinical accounts as well as in interviews with oocyte recipients, it is problematized in the case of freezers. For example, Maria reflects upon the oocytes that she has left in the cryopreservation tank: "It's a little weird, because they're not babies, but they're still my eggs, so it's like you don't want anyone hurting them, kind of, but then they're really eggs. So it's kind of like, you know. Like, really, they're not going to feel pain—so it's just sort of like—it's a weird thing, but I might be willing to do something with them eventually."

Affects of love and attachment work to produce very gendered understandings of oocytes and make oocytes appear more like babies. In the case of Tina, she recalls how a major hurricane in New York City worried her while she traveled to London for business: "Oh, my God, my babies! [laughter]. Once I had them frozen, that was it. I was done. I would just write a check out, whatever. Bring out the credit card every year when I got the bill. So I was glad that somebody was thinking to airlift these things! But the eggs were fine." Meanwhile, Annette is more explicit in what she says about her eggs in the freezer: "Yeah. I think of them as my potential children, and I think it would be hard to discard them. So we'll have to see." This intimate relationship between eggs and future babies is echoed in the Danish bioethical deliberations, in which egg cells are positioned as an integral part of a woman's identity: "Women quite naturally consider their eggs as an integral part of their body" (Danish Council on Ethics 2012). Here, oocytes appear as microcosms of individual women's identities. This is in sharp contrast to the understanding of sperm as naturally flowing from men's bodies and in no way representative of men's identities.

Of course, this link between oocytes and babies may not be surprising. In the Danish flyer *Egg Donors Are Needed—Is That YOU?*, a small, fully grown baby rests in an adult female hand, looking past the viewer.[14] The QR code is positioned between this white baby's hands, perhaps enabling the viewer to get more information or even to imagine this child as having a very specific, own genetic makeup. The main text is written inside what could be an egg-shaped circle and juxtaposed on top of another similar circle. The background, surrounded by the color green, works to make oocyte providing appear hopeful, as green is an emotionally positive color, perhaps even connoting a sense of nature of sorts. Meanwhile, dandelion seeds, known to travel relatively far distances (here having an uncanny resemblance to the egg), are vaguely represented in the background of the main text, the language of which suggests that the need for oocyte providers can be positioned as an opportunity for them to give a "beautiful gift," to allow someone else "the chance to become a mother." Neither the egg provider nor the recipient is present, nor are the necessary treatments (needles, hormones, extraction, medication).

In sharp contrast to the notion of eggs as babies or microcosms of self, oocytes, as related in interviews with Danish women who travel to Spain, have microscopic potentiality—"tiny cells," genetic and necessary "spare parts." The fact that oocytes are repeatedly described by recipients as tiny has the effect of making oocytes appear as just a minor technology on a long list of reproductive interventions, similar to hormone treatments, pregnancy, birth, and breastfeeding. This is also, as evident in Kroløkke (2014), the case with Nete. Here, medical history necessitates egg providing. Consequently, the provider oocyte is akin to the long list of medical treatments that Nete has already undergone. In what Nete refers to as "a stranger's egg," the oocyte is a simple and tiny part of the reproductive cycle. In fact, pregnancy and childbirth are the determining factors that re-naturalize Nete's motherhood.

Nete: Of course they [the babies] should know about it but also, we do not want to make a bigger deal out of it because it has never been that to us. I think the difference between being an egg donor and sperm donor is huge.

Interviewer: How is it different?

Nete: It has to do with the fact that the pregnancy lasts for nine months and that if we had used a sperm donor, then Will [Nete's husband] would not have had any connection to it. And I really do think that I have. Even though this is a stranger's egg but really it is such a tiny, tiny, tiny . . . and then, from then on it is only me.

Will: We are used to using spare parts [laughs]. (Kroløkke 2014: 66)

Not only recipients but also providers echo the idea that oocytes are positioned as "simply" necessary parts. The Irish IVF Clinic, which is labeled "Simply Egg Donation," refers to recipients being given the choice of two Ukrainian providers.[15] To global egg providers such as Tracy, "simply" refers to the oocyte as being nothing but an "ingredient" in a cake: "Egg donation is just like borrowing an ingredient for a cake. It doesn't make the cake, but is an essential part of it." Similarly, Lucy notes that she is "loaning a bit of my body for a short period of time," and Lotte agrees when she says, "I am not giving a baby away to a stranger; I'm merely giving them 'cells' (so to speak) that have the possibility of producing a baby. I mean, let's face it, little eggs are not something we get emotionally attached to! So why not give them to someone that needs them?" In the words of Keri, "It was just there, a tiny bit of DNA that I sure wasn't going to use."

The notion of egg cells as "tiny parts" or "little eggs" is also central in the marketing material. Here, an aesthetic and visual outcome is reproduced, in which healthy, beautiful babies and happy recipient mothers are the result of IVF. The clinical discourses shift from the egg as a carrier of various predispositions to the importance of pregnancy (shared nutrients) and the immunological protection that the pregnant woman (the intended mother) grants the developing baby (Kroløkke 2014). So this becomes an "own" baby through doing reproductive, somatic work (pregnancy and birth), as well as affective labor (hope and desire).

The move from "tiny cells" to "own babies" is inherent in the implantation procedures. Here, narratives surrounding visualization technologies transform provider oocytes into "own" future babies. In the Spanish clinic, recipients intensely watch the TV monitor displaying the fertilized oocyte, located in the petri dish, labeled with the intended mother's name. The fertilized oocyte is now carried by the biologist from the reproductive lab into the operating theater, where it is ready for implantation. The fact that recipients can see the fertilized oocyte is important. First, it enables them to see the fertilized oocyte "returned," marking a moment in which reproductive cells become "own" future babies. Tine notes, "In reality, [they felt like they were mine] when I saw [what was happening onscreen]. You see that there are two . . . two oocytes or two . . . they are not simply oocytes. One had six cells and the other seven cells, which was great. At that point I felt . . . they are mine. They really have to develop. Now I am going to take care of you two that are now inside of me." Moreover, it deprioritizes "conception" and re-naturalizes "implantation" as an enhanced, new, mediated moment of conception. It testifies to the importance of what Rose (2007) refers to as a molecular gaze. Or as noted by the Danish fertility traveler Lars, who, in going to Prague together with his wife for treatment, expresses that visualization technologies grant him an ability to take up a gendered masculine role: "This is the closest I get to impregnat[ing] my wife."

The idea of "own" babies is clearly choreographed in the clinical practice to fit parental intent (Thompson 2005). The notion of "own" unfolds in an entanglement with love, hope, and happiness combined with maternal behaviors (a focus on healthy eating, a healthy pregnancy, etc.). Moreover, in the Spanish clinic, "own" unfolds once a provider has been selected, while "own" in the case of Line, a fertility traveler to Spain, occurs at the moment "when the body accepts the fertilized egg."

The notion of an own child, however, is also the product of a significant economic investment, or as argued by Thea who has chosen to freeze a cycle of her eggs, "A lot of my friends here spend ten thousand dollars on a vacation, without thinking about it, every year, twice a year. . . . Look at how much we spend on rent, car parking, clothing . . . when you add it all up, the actual egg freezing is so cheap, because it gives you this . . . people use the word 'insurance.' I don't. The way I see it is, it gives you such happiness later on, that you could have." When "own" entangles with happiness, it makes freezing a legitimate, even inexpensive choice. As argued by Ahmed (2010) in her cultural critique of happiness as a compulsory affect, happiness makes certain routes understandable, even legitimate and natural. This is similarly present in the observations undertaken during the "Take Back Your Fertility" seminar in London, where narratives on future happiness are situated in close proximity to reproductive control and gender equality simultaneously upholding motherhood as central to a woman's sense of accomplishment and psychological well-being.

While oocytes are tiny cells to the providers and the recipients, they are clearly embedded within a transnational economy in hope (Franklin 1997). To Tina, her frozen oocytes signal reassurance: "But just the fact that I had these eggs frozen somewhere made me very comfortable. It was very reassuring for me, because otherwise it was just like this mad race to find a partner to have a baby with, and I'm like, 'I don't care!' I mean, I could find a partner, I am dating somebody, but now it doesn't matter whether I get married to him." Meanwhile, in the clinic, hope is displayed in the photos of healthy, happy-looking babies, as well as clinical success rates promising patients a 60–70 percent success rate.[16] As noted by Rose (2007) and Novas (2006), hope is both individualized and collectivized. While hope is individualized and made into a particular woman's chance at motherhood or a child, hope is also collectivized in the more generic marketing material, enabling the older Northern European women who can afford it a chance at motherhood, as well as in clinical practices in which personal aspirations, clinical success rates, and professional ambitions all intertwine in the name of hope.

In this third analytical incision, I have illustrated how oocytes become "tiny cells" (when donated or received), microcosms of self (in ethical accounts as well as when frozen), and future "own" babies (when fertilized, implanted, or frozen). In the clinical practices, clinicians ensure emotional and physical distance between providers and recipients: not only do they often enter different parts of the clinic (even completely different buildings in some cases), the oocyte is also clearly marked and labeled in terms of its reproductive path, ensuring a particular directionality that de-emphasizes where the oocyte came from (frequently from poorer women) and naturalizes where the oocyte is going (frequently to older, more financially stable women from the North).

Imagined Reproductive, Rightful Bodies

> You are both beautiful, amazing people. I really wish you the best, and I hope that the process works for you and you get exactly what you have been dreaming of. (Tanya, egg provider)

Love and beauty circulate to produce an understanding of transnational fertility treatments as a rightful and pan-humanitarian act. Not only are recipient couples frequently imagined to be "beautiful," "amazing," and "loving," egg providers are also imagined to be "young," "altruistic," and "empowered." In this section, I turn to the ways that providers and recipients are imagined in clinical and personal accounts. As noted by Berglund and Lundin (2012) in their work on transnational organ transfers, recipients spend a lot of time imagining the organ provider. I agree and extend this to egg providers, who, in their accounts, similarly envision particular types of normative recipient bodies (well-adjusted, happy, loving, successful, and frequently heterosexual). However, I first discuss the ways that the ideal oocyte provider rhetorically, materially, and in and through affects comes to matter. I then turn to the ways that the oocyte provider is constructed as an informational and bland reproductive body as well as, in cases of egg freezing, an ageless and rightful body.

Informational and Bland Reproductive Bodies

In the Spanish clinical setting, two nurses match providers and recipients daily. Their workstation is in a separate building from where the international patients arrive. Unlike the larger clinic this building is frequented by the providers, yet it is unknown to the recipients. Located within a brief two-minute walk from the clinic's impressive main entrance, the front doors to this building are hardly noticeable, as one must walk down a few stairs to get into the more humble offices. It contrasts starkly with the shiny, new, steel-looking large clinic that is busy with fertility doctors, thirteen international coordinators, and international patients.

As I arrive, the nurses are busy scrutinizing provider and recipient photos, comparing and contrasting phenotypes, taking particular notice of eye color. Today, their first task is to match a German recipient woman with frozen oocytes already available in the clinic. This kind of work, the nurses say, requires them not only to *find* the best provider, but also to *imagine* what the future child might look like. Eye color is the most important trait, the nurses tell me. While I know, from information given in interviews and conversations with the recipients, that a Spanish provider is expected and desired, the nurses de-emphasize nationality and instead focus on physical similarity of the provider and recipient. The green-eyed recipient must be matched with the green-eyed provider, they say, unless her husband has brown eyes "of course." Having a number of frozen oocytes available at the clinic makes matching easier, and on this day, the nurses happily find a "perfect" provider fairly easily—one who not only physically matches the recipient as far as colors are concerned but who also has a great record of high-quality eggs, the nurses inform me, defined by them as a previously successful provider.

In the Spanish clinical setting, the optimal provider is one who has been previously successful and who blends with the recipient to successfully produce an "own" child. Similarly, the Czech medical tourism director notes that the ideal provider is "so bland or so average that she does not stand out." When I ask what "bland" means, he defines it as "average Czech appearance," which he says means white skin, average intelligence, standard height and weight. Similarly, the international coordinators emphasize blandness, but they recount numerous recipient requests for provider attractiveness, intelligence, and educational background. Jane, a Danish woman on her way to Spain, actively resists blandness in desiring an attractive provider. As an attractive and professionally successful woman in her mid-forties, Jane stresses that attractiveness and IQ matter. However, Jane feels reassured that the clinical attentiveness to her own appearance resembles a privileging of sameness: "They do pay a lot of attention to height, size, and colors. And it is probably quite important to me because I can feel that it is quality, that it is alright," she says.

In the clinical discourses, provider and recipient bodies are informational bodies. John and Kari have been given basic information about their chosen provider and note several points of similarity with Kari. Not only do the two women seemingly share an interest in gymnastics and dance, their similarities extend to a shared biology of sorts:

Kali: Yes. It is kind of crazy. We were told that . . . Well, we had to tell them about how we look—nothing about hobbies or anything, only looks. So the donor will be blonde, light skin and green eyes. She is 168 [cm].

John: No, 165 cm and 58 kilo. With a BMI similar to us, right? Twenty-eight years of age.

Kali: Like me and she already has a child. And she is a rhythmic gymnast—a gym teacher. (Kroløkke 2014: 65)

The informational body is coded according to phenotypes and BMI, but it is also understood within a larger context of geopolitics and religion in particular. In the stories of recipients traveling to Spain, Catholic cultural values are positioned in close proximity to the presumed Spanish providers, which makes going to Spain appear like a "natural" choice. In the case of Mike and Ruby, for example, going to Spain from Ireland is in large part due to presumed cultural and religious similarities: "Culturally we are quite similar. Catholic country. Similar outlook on life, so I know a lot about Spain. I don't know anything about the Ukraine, and that was kind of the other option we had," Mike says. While Mike and Ruby also make reference to Ruby's "dark colors" throughout the interview, they repeatedly mention a similarity in "outlook on life" as critical in their choice to go to Spain (Kroløkke 2014).

To fertility travelers, the informational body extends to other local women who become stand-ins for the imagined provider. Rita traveled to Barcelona and comments on the Spanish women present in the waiting room: "None of them looked like they were dying of starvation or oppressed or anything. I remember one who came swaying through the waiting room with hips, big breasts, and the whole nine yards, and the entire waiting room was like [shows her mouth dropping and she laughs]." Here, hips and big breasts combined with a particular posture ("swaying") and a healthy weight signals empowerment and makes fertility and equality go hand in hand ("none of them looked like they were dying of starvation or oppressed"). Similarly, the Czech women that Anne meets in Prague put her at ease: "I just walked around and looked at all the women. Wow . . . you are all so beautiful. It was really fantastic. You are all smiling. You are really nice. Great . . . give me your eggs."

In these tales, reproductive bodies are bland as well as informational. Whereas provider bodies, in the clinical practices, are stand-in genetic material, in the cultural imaginary of recipients and in the meetings that take place between recipients and other local women, they are attractive, sensuous, and feminine reproductive bodies that embody altruism through smiling and particular body types (the voluptuous body). Thus, I turn now to the making of exotic, ageless, and rightful reproductive bodies.

Exotic, Ageless and Rightful Reproductive Bodies

Going beyond the bland and informational body, interviews with fertility travelers and freezers suggest the emergence of an exotic, ageless, and rightful reproductive body. In the material, Spanish ova and Western European "quality" stick together, while egg freezing becomes the Botox of fertility,[17] a reinvigoration of the reproductive aging body.

In the case of Spain, the imagined provider entangles with an attractive Mediterranean ideal (Kroløkke 2014). Several of the recipients naturalize their decision to go to Spain through a narrative of resemblance coupled with exoticism: "Frequently people have asked me whether or not I come from Spain because of my colors and stuff like that but I am thinking . . . but in summers I can get quite tanned and then I have kind of dark eyebrows, and when my hair gets light in the summer, it's obviously a little Spanish in color," Jane says. To Kali, resemblance extends beyond appearance to hobbies and general outlook on life, an outgoing type of people as well as a proclivity toward a particular type of music and dance, defined by her as "Latin" music and rhythm:

> Kali: Yes also the samba community. It is Latin music you play, right? So that environment . . . combined with having to go abroad. There haven't been many Russians or Finns [in her previous community and in her relationship with individuals that speak Spanish], so maybe that is why I associate it a little bit with dance. Very alive and outgoing perhaps . . . so of course we have really considered it a lot. I mean I have . . .
>
> John: You have [laughs].
>
> Kali: I mean—this thing with dance. I have really thought about that. I mean now that we are talking about it . . . I have thought about this thing with the very alive, outgoing people. You really have to believe in what you pass on to the child in some way or another, right?
>
> John: But it is also what you sort of imagine—there is more life gest, isn't there? I mean—south of the Alps. There is more sun down there in comparison to Helsinki or wherever. There [Helsinki] it is cold and people are pale and it is, you know, a little . . .
>
> Kali: Just like the rest of us [laughs]. (Kroløkke 2014: 64)

In this "South of the Alps" narrative, having Spanish roots (and rhythm) creates a desirable procreation story. Dance comes to exemplify the exotic, while it also transcends cultural differences (now grouped into the category of foreign dance) and differences between women (in this case between Kali and the provider) (Kroløkke 2014). While Kali's imagined provider is made to appear exotic, she is also situated as more similar to Kali than an imagined Finnish provider (Kroløkke 2014). Franklin et al. describe the traffic between similarity and exotic difference in regard to the consumption of globalized consumer goods: "By consuming global products, the western subject and the exotic other are thus reaffirmed, even as such a dichotomy is apparently transcended by the appeal to a universal global culture" (Franklin et al. 2000: 104). Similarly, in the case of Kali and John, the choice to go to Spain is reaffirmed through Kali's own participation in what is constructed as another exotic community, the samba community, thus making a trip "South of the Alps" a natural and more likely reproductive choice.

The Danish recipients imagine a friendly, outgoing, and even temperamental Spanish culture as desirable. Yet, as echoed in Kroløkke (2014), the exoticness of Spain is contained in numerous ways as well. For instance, Jane repeatedly mentions the importance of provider attractiveness, while Rita recounts stressing the provider's intellectual abilities and recounts her dialogue with the female doctor at the Barcelona clinic: "I just wanted to know that she had as good chances as possible at becoming as intelligent as possible, so I did ask, if they had the same thing with medical students that we have here—that a lot of medical students give sperm but they said that they didn't. Then, we really looked seriously at each other, and I think she as a doctor kept that in mind when she selected," Rita says. Where intellectual abilities are important to Rita, Jane comments that her boyfriend has a very high IQ, and so she privileges a certain degree of attractiveness: "I do know that it is not important what the child looks like, but of course you do wonder about it. I do hope that it is not a totally ugly donor. It is horrible to say, but I do. But the most important thing is of course health. But I do of course think . . . How about those genes?"

The idea of an exotic Spain is managed in other ways as well. Notably, recipients imagine the provider as a caring individual, while clinical discourses work to substantiate this imagination. On the website of one of the leading Spanish fertility clinics, the providers are depicted as young and attractive, with white, olive skin and brown eyes and hair.[18] In the case of the female egg provider, she wears a white strap top and a pleasant smile, and looks directly and invitingly at the viewer. Both providers embody an urban aesthetic of sorts. This urban and pan-European appearance reinforces the idea that the providers could be from anywhere in Europe (Kroløkke 2014). It minimizes differences and reinstates the notion that providers happily and willingly give (not sell) their biogenetic substances. The images of the potential providers are gendered, classed, and heterosexed: they reveal attractive individuals, possibly university students, and by engaging the viewer's gaze, these providers appear socially competent (Kroløkke 2015b).

The argument put forward here is that these recipient imaginations work to make oocytes appear as global fluids that naturally move between women that are perhaps differently aged but similarly empowered. The rhetoric of gifting creates an idea of a globalized, shared femininity—uniting women everywhere in the world as providers and recipients—united in a naturalized desire to have children and experience the joy of motherhood. The imagined differences are made to appear both acceptable and even exotic, enabling an intimate sharing of what Franklin et al. frame as "the embodiment of flows that unite inner and outer within a set of mutually dependent systems" (Franklin et al. 2000: 127). Anonymity encourages recipients to imagine other women as potential providers, while in the case of global egg providers, recipients pick the provider of their choice (along with photos and detailed descriptions). Meanwhile, providers specify their desired destination. Mobility is embedded in these transactions, both in the tendency to emphasize a particular directionality (travel to new destinations, imagined reproductive futures) as well as in the ability to arrest reproductive futurity (egg freezing), situating the quest for a child within a grand narrative of mobility.

While recipients imagine providers as informational and exotic bodies, the imagined recipient is depicted in egg provider essays and in the clinical marketing material as a good and rightful person. The ideal recipient is someone who has undergone various unsuccessful IVF treatments, replacing provider reproductive work with recipient dreams for maternity. The clinical websites support this understanding of the attractive recipient woman. Featuring translations in English, German, French, and Italian, the website of one prominent Spanish clinic displays a young and seemingly single, attractive woman who looks directly at the viewer and smiles. When clicking on the language, the text ("I wish to fulfill my dream") stays the same, but the female photo changes to match imagined racialized and nationalized women. In the case of the German site, the featured recipient woman is blonde, while different imagined recipient women with dark hair are present on the French and Spanish sites, for example.[19] This image of the ideal recipient is also recognizable in global egg providers' accounts. Marcia, for instance, who traveled to California and Barbados, says, "I hope and pray that you fall pregnant, and have healthy, happy children. I know that you will be phenomenal, fun, loving parents. I cannot imagine the pain and heartache that you have been through. I know that you are amazing, strong, successful people who deserve all the happiness in the world. If you ever need me for anything at all, don't be shy to ask. I wish you both everything of the best. Love and blessings, your donor." Similarly, Emma, who went to California, comments upon the recipients' pain and desire when she says, "I read my recipients' first essay, where they informed me why they are going through the process. I shed a tear and went to bed." In these two accounts, the imagined recipients are not only "deserving," they are described by the providers as "successful," "amazing," "strong," "fun," and "loving" people.

The providers know very little about the recipients, yet affects of love and happiness work to make the recipients appear "worthy" and "rightful" individuals. In her account of the imagined recipient couple, Jeff and Bill, Lara recounts her connection with them that is partially, at least, due to their writing skills in general and their grammar in particular. Love re-naturalizes Jeff and Bill's desire for fatherhood: "The couple in question, Jeff and Bill, sent me a heart-melting introduction full of compassion, kindness and the most beautiful enthusiasm about the prospect of becoming fathers. (And to top it all off, their grammar was perfect!) I instantly felt a connection with them and was very honored to become part of their story. In the lead-up to the donation, we shared letters that would have me gushing over the phone to mum, "They sound SO nice! And they know how to use semicolons!" Love, not gender, is what is required to make a family successful, Lara purports. The fact that this recipient couple is articulate and uses proper English does something: knowing how to use semicolons not only makes for smooth readings, it also reinforces the idea of this recipient couple as educated, middle-class, and by extension rightful parents.

In total, the previous two subsections have demonstrated some of the ways that recipients and providers daydream and engage in the production of normative, rightful reproductive bodies. When viewed as global fluids, eggs contribute to the making of bland, informational, and even exotic reproductive bodies. Ice equals stasis, yet it assists in the production of ageless reproductive bodies. These narratives, coupled with the clinical practices, engage with a grand narrative of mobility, vitality (fertility) and young bodies, turning recipients into good, loving, and rightful reproductive bodies.

From Waste to Entrepreneurial Value

I have illustrated how oocytes move from being excess and wasteful material to becoming investments, gifts, commodities, tiny cells, and "own" babies, while also contributing to the making of bland, informational, exotic, and rightful reproductive bodies. In this concluding section, I will show how disentangling eggs from innate biological matter leads to an understanding of eggs as having distributive, regenerative, speculative, and entrepreneurial value. It involves a "transformation in kinds of value" (Waldby and Mitchell 2006: 114) and illustrates how the opposition between what gets constructed as valuable and value*less* is misleading (Waldby and Mitchell 2006).

The distributive value of oocytes is obtained at the point of extraction. Up until then, the egg belongs to the provider, and she can withdraw from the exchange at any point. Upon extraction, eggs become mobile and, once frozen, potential global commodities—much like sperm. Eggs are either handpicked from one specific provider for a specific recipient (in the case of Global Egg Donors) or from a larger group of providers, re-activating geopolitical imaginations of more generic, attractive Spanish and Czech providers. While Spanish eggs gain distributive value as empowered, quality, and Western matter, Czech providers are innately friendly and attractive, and they are also in the business of producing desirable genetic material. Meanwhile, recipients' or egg freezers' own, yet aging, eggs have little, if any, distributive value.

The redistribution of eggs from one woman to another is made to appear natural, even rewarding. Hence, global egg providers express pride and thankfulness for having been chosen as a provider. As noted by Tracy, who went to Mexico, "I have been chosen not even a month after I had joined the clinic. It really is a bit of an ego boost. 'What? Somebody chose ME above all these other beautiful donors? Somebody wants ME to help them to have a baby?' What an honor and a privilege!" This sentiment is echoed in other accounts: "A couple had chosen me from all the profiles. What an honor that my eggs were the ones that they wanted to make their child! This feeling, that an unknown couple, somewhere out in this big world, chose me to help them! And on top of that, they wanted me to come to Cancun, Mexico!" Keri, who traveled to India, says, "The feeling that you get that somebody out there wants your eggs is indescribable! You kind of catch yourself saying, why me, I'm so ordinary?! My self-esteem shot through the roof." Eggs achieve distributive value through a series of events: providers are chosen, then eggs are matured (escaping the zero value of a menstrual flow), monitored (on the ultrasound machine), extracted (in the clinical setting), fertilized, and later implanted in the recipient woman (with the assistance of a full bladder and ultrasound technology).

Eggs gain regenerative value through the promises of extended fertility, as well as a healthy, aging body. As argued by Waldby and Cooper (2008), reproductive exchanges involve an attunement to the body's ability to regenerate itself, but it is also contingent upon reproductive technologies, clinical infrastructures, and a pool of reproductive workers frequently located in the third world and in the South. To the infertile and older Northern European woman, who travels to Spain for treatment, eggs are a "shot of fertility" afforded by a younger, empowered Spanish woman. In this case, younger eggs restore older women's fertility and sensuality, while in the case of freezing, they arrest women's fertility and aging while extending the allure of compulsory heterosexual coupledom.

Although not present in this empirical material, eggs also gain regenerative value when they entangle with the stem cell industries and when they hold the promise of future cures (Waldby and Cooper 2008)—or, as evident here, when they are positioned as material that regenerates multiple times throughout a woman's reproductive life. In the case of Spanish providers or global egg providers, they entangle with notions of plentitude and spare eggs.

In the encounter between freezing technologies, the fertility industry, and a population of women that can afford it, eggs gain speculative and entrepreneurial value as bioassets. Freezing arrests the generative capacities of eggs in time and space. Its promise is still somewhat speculative, however. Not only may the success rate of live births with thirty-eight-year-old frozen eggs be approximately 70 percent per thirty eggs frozen,[20] freezers may also have few mature oocytes or may in fact choose never to thaw or use them. Moreover, the speculative value extends beyond the immediate fertility potential to the dating and romantic potential (Carroll and Kroløkke 2017). Lea illustrates the latter point when, in reference to having thirty-two eggs on ice and to her status as a single woman dating in New York City, she says, "People [men] often ask me, like, 'Oh, do you have eggs?' and it's like, 'I do have eggs!'" The "I do have eggs" statement reveals how

Lea reinstates herself not only as a potential future mother but also, importantly, as "wife potential." Meanwhile, eggs gain entrepreneurial value when egg providers use their potent eggs to engage in the mobility of financially better-off recipients and travel to see the world.

To draw the different empirical material together, I have discussed how eggs gain (new) meanings throughout their extraction, industrialization, commodification, vitrification, and consumption processes. As already shown, what may have the appearance of zero value to the providers gains distributive value to the recipients, speculative value in the case of freezers, and entrepreneurial value to the global egg providers who use their oocytes to see the world. Meanwhile, the economic exchange and somatic work that go into the making of good eggs is turned into a globalized femininity, in which altruism and motherhood become cemented as universally attractive, as well as innately shared.

Notes

The analysis in this chapter relies on previously published material in Kroløkke 2014, "West Is Best: Affective Assemblages and Spanish Oöcytes," *European Journal of Women's Studies* 21(1): 57–71, and Kroløkke, C. 2015a. "Have Eggs,Will Travel: The Ethics of Global Egg Donation." *Journal of Somatechnics: Special Issue on Medical Travel and Bioethics* 5(1): 12–31, and in Kroløkke, C. 2015b. "The Golden Egg: The Business of Making Motherhood through Egg Donation." In *The Motherhood Business: Consumption, Communication and Privilege,* edited by A. Demo, J. Borda, and C. Kroløkke, 28–51, Tuscaloosa: University of Alabama Press.

1. The price of a round of egg providing varies, but in this clinic the starting price is €7,000 (equivalent to US$8,200). Yet, as revealed in the interviews with recipients, as hotel and flight expenses were added on, the price was frequently close to €10,000 (equivalent to US$12,000). For an example of the price see IVI, "In Vitro Fertilisation," https://ivi-fertility.com/ivf-invitro-price/ (retrieved October 2017).
2. Because interview studies are exempt from internal review board (IRB) approval in Denmark, I have followed the guidelines stipulated by the European Science Foundation (ESF) on good research practice. This entails that informed consent, anonymity, and privacy have been given and all participants have been met with openness and integrity. For more information on the ESF guidelines see ALLEA—All European Academies, "The European Code of Conduct for Research Intregrity, Revised Edition," European Commission, 2017, http://ec.europa.eu/research/participants/data/ref/h2020/other/hi/h2020-ethics_code-of-conduct_en.pdf (retrieved January 2016).
3. I carried out observations in a Barcelona clinic during three separate

trips of approximately one week each throughout 2012. The chosen clinic is popular with international patients and has subsidiaries in all major Spanish cities, as well as a presence in a total of ten different countries (Argentina, Brazil, Chile, Mexico, Panama, India, United Arab Emirates, Italy, Portugal, and Spain). During the fieldwork, I observed in the operating theater; participated in first consultations with German, Dutch, English, and Danish couples; talked with the international coordinators; and observed in the matching department.

4. Today, egg freezing is an important service provided by fertility clinics located in metropolitan areas in the United Kingdom and United States. Whereas a round of egg freezing approximately costs US$10,000 in New York, an egg freezer in London must expect to pay approximately 5,000 pounds (equivalent to approximately US$4,000), excluding various costs associated with medication, blood tests, monitoring, and health checks. Additionally, egg freezers will have to pay for future IVF (not frequently included in the egg-freezing fees). For more detailed information concerning the costs associated with the London Women's Clinic in the United Kingdom, see the London Women's Clinic website: http://www.londonwomensclinic.com/fertility-services/how-much-is-egg-freezing.htm (retrieved October 2017).
5. The empirical material includes a total of thirty-six interviews (twenty interviews with Danish fertility travelers, sixteen interviews with U.S. freezers) as well as a range of conversations with foreign couples present in the Barcelona clinic. Whereas Danish fertility travelers were interviewed in a location of their choice, all other interviews were carried out in the clinics.
6. The empirical material also includes interviews with five traveling providers and analyses of forty-two travel accounts, written and submitted to the agency Global Egg Donors. Global Egg Donors is an intermediary agency that enables egg providers to stipulate their destination choice, while recipients can read about all the available providers, see photos of them and sometimes photos of their children, and request a particular provider. I interviewed the director of Global Egg Donors and received access to the online egg-provider profiles, along with the travel essays that each provider must submit upon ending her provider trip. The travel essays varied in length, from half a page to several pages of writing plus photos. My interviews with global egg providers were conducted over the phone and took place while doing fieldwork at a leading fertility clinic in Barbados.
7. To understand how oocytes are mediated in the marketing material, the empirical material includes select campaigns on oocyte providing and freezing, as well as the overall developments that have occurred within Danish bioethical discussions and legislation throughout the time period of 2010–16.
8. "Smart women freeze!" https://www.eggbanxx.com/ (retrieved June 2016). Located in Manhattan, Eggbanxx combines a network of doc-

tors with a payment plan, which they say makes egg freezing simple and easy.

9. Eggbanxx argues that women who choose to freeze are looking to *maximize* their chances of having a *healthy* baby. See more at https://www.eggbanxx.com/ (retrieved June 2016).
10. Copenhagen Fertility Center engages the potential client with the promise of swift treatment. Available at: http://www.copenhagenfertilitycenter.com/nyheder/ingen-ventetid-paa-aegdonation-hos-os-.htm (retrieved June 2016).
11. This statement is available on the Global Egg Donors home page and also appears in an interview with the owner: http://www.globaleggdonors.com/donors (retrieved June 2017).
12. More information about the SIMS IVF program including their collaborations with Eastern European clinics can be found on the clinic's website: http://www.eggdonation.ie/home/simply-keyid.1195.html (retrieved April 2018).
13. The empirical material includes visits to three different fertility clinics in Alicante, Spain. Alicante is another well-known Spanish tourist destination with direct, inexpensive flight connections from Northern Europe.
14. The visual is present at the Bliv Æddonor "become an egg donor" site: http://www.blivaegdonor.dk/ (retrieved May 2017).
15. More information on egg donation can be found on the SIMS website: http://www.eggdonation.ie/home/simply-keyid.1195.html (retrieved April 2018).
16. http://www.copenhagenfertilitycenter.com/nyheder/ingen-ventetid-paa-aegdonation-hos-os-.htm (retrieved June 2016).
17. The article titled "Women Can't Botox Their Ovaries" critiques the positioning of egg freezing as a reproductive technique employed to postpone motherhood: S. Fenton, "'Women Can't Botox Their Ovaries' and the Best Time to Give Birth is 25, Warns Fertility Expert," The Independent, June 15, 2016, http://www.independent.co.uk/life-style/health-and-families/health-news/you-cant-botox-your-ovaries-fertility-expert-warns-amid-concerns-over-young-women-delaying-pregnancy-a7083091.html (retrieved June 2016).
18. The Spanish clinic IVI recruits egg providers through their website such as evident on this page: https://www.ivi.es/donantes/ (retrieved March 2015).
19. Whereas the IVI provider website is directed towards younger Western European women, the website targeting recipients portrays more mature women: https://www.ivi-fertility.com/de/?_ga=1.58147880.386039902.1465894014 (retrieved March 2015).
20. The Northern California Fertility Center stipulates that successful IVF following egg freezing is highly dependent on the number of eggs frozen and the age at which eggs are retrieved and vitrified. See more at http://www.ncfmc.com/fertility-preservation/egg-freezing/ (retrieved June 2016).

Chapter 4

Placentas
From Waste to Regeneration

> "We were petrified that they were going to realize that we had it," says the mother, who is still too nervous about the placenta-snatching to go on the record with her name. The placenta was important to her. She wanted to eat it (Sauerwein 2014).

The headline "Mom Smuggles Placenta after Hospital Refused to Release It" sounds like a reproductive cover-up operation, where the placenta is not merely afterbirth matter but an "own" healing bioproduct full of potentiality—in this case vitamins and minerals. This Texas mom was "forced," we are told, to "smuggle" the placenta out of the hospital. While she is positioned as "exhausted" from just having given birth, she is simultaneously "petrified" and too "nervous" to have her name on record. In contrast, her husband jumps into action and succeeds in getting the placenta, placing it in a cooler and passing it on to the individual undertaking the encapsulation process, thereby saving the placenta ("we got the placenta"). In this chapter I show how placentas come to matter in concrete practices, in marketing material, in and through metaphors, and in mediated accounts. I first briefly describe the placenta's physical attributes and then present the assemblage of material that goes into these placenta tales.

Attached to the wall of the uterus, the placenta is a reproductive organ that develops during pregnancy, weighing an average of six hundred grams, measuring fifteen to twenty centimeters in diameter with a thickness of two to two and a half centimeters. Frequently referred to as "afterbirth," it is also known in Danish as "mother cake." Whereas "afterbirth" refers to the fact that the placenta arrives after the baby, "placenta" is Latin for "uterine cake," making reference to the placenta's round, flat cake-like appearance, as well as gendered understandings of the womb as an oven: "The placenta had acted like a raising agent, allowing the 'dough' to take shape" (Gelis 1996 167). The placenta protects the fetus and, through hormone production and waste management, nourishes the baby during pregnancy. Delivered fifteen to sixty minutes after the birth of the baby, it is uniquely positioned in terms of its materiality, produced and intended for a very specific purpose, belonging to more than one body at a time and sharing 100 percent of the developing baby's DNA (Passariello 1994).

Placenta Sites

The material that goes into this chapter includes interviews, photographic material, marketing campaigns, debates, and mediated accounts, as well as TV documentaries on placenta consumption as a new trend among new mothers in Denmark and the United Kingdom.[1] Participating in a cross-cultural research project that involved interview participants from the United States and Denmark,[2] I interviewed Danish women who had consumed the placenta after birth (whether as encapsulated pills, raw, or cooked). I visited one placenta preparer and spoke with Danish midwives who receive and handle placentas after birth.[3] One of the midwives contributed a series of photos from a Danish public birthing clinic documenting the ways that the placenta moves from the birthing body to the hospital's refrigerated waste container.[4] Two other interviewees contributed photos of their placenta consumption choices. Moreover, to understand how placenta consumption is debated, I put together an archive of UK and Danish media accounts.[5] Because the placenta acquires value beyond the intimate sphere of the individual birthing woman and crosses human and animal borders, I tracked how human and also porcine placentas become raw resources in the Asian pharmaceutical and cosmetic industry. I visited one Japanese pharmaceutical company that uses human and porcine placentas in the development of anti-aging and whitening cosmetic products, and I researched the ways that Danish pig farmers collect porcine afterbirth and refrigerate it[6] before another company picks up the afterbirth for processing and circulation into the Asian pharmaceutical and cosmetic industry.[7] Finally, I turn to the ways that the emergent stem cell industry in the United States markets placenta storage as a health investment in order to gain the promise of future treatment.[8]

The empirical material comes from four very different geopolitical locations: Denmark, the United Kingdom, the United States, and Japan. Whereas the European Union today is one of the most legally restrictive regions with regard to the use and distribution, processing, and marketing of human and animal placentas, in Japan the collection, processing, and export of human and animal placenta-based products are fully legal. In the case of human cosmetic placenta products, however, the products are first exported abroad and then imported back to Japan as a prescription drug, through the authorization and licenses of Japanese doctors. The Japanese human placenta cosmetic products are sold in Russia and throughout Asia, and due to the fact that cosmetic companies in the United States can use any ingredient and market it without prior approval from the U.S. Food and Drug Administration (FDA),[9] human placenta cosmetic products, including Japanese products, are also sold in the United States. Because legal and ethical regulations are important, I briefly turn in the material to the European Food Safety Authority (EFSA) regulations, and I focus on the 2014 decision to classify placenta food as a "novel food"[10] and the debates that arose in its wake. Meanwhile, placenta cord banking is especially prominent in the United States. This cross-cultural collection of empirical material is by no means exhaustive. However, it does suggest that placentas cross national, bodily, personal, legal, ethical, and commercial borders as multi-potent matter.

Placenta Tales

In various tales and legends, the placenta takes on different meanings. It has been cast as the child's mother, its younger or older sister/brother, as well as its double (a second child), frequently positioned within existing kin relationships. Outlining the historical significance and different cultural understandings of the placenta, Long (1963) points to a vast array of cross-cultural meanings and understandings: the placenta is situated as having a soul, rooting and protecting the child, for example, yet also gaining medicinal value—it can be cooked, dried and consumed to promote fertility, or, in the case of Austria and parts of Italy, it becomes a possible cure for epilepsy (Long 1963). Similarly, Passariello (1994) notes how the placenta has been understood as the newborn's twin and the mother of the child, while Kroløkke (2011) illustrates how the placenta is mediated during the prenatal ultrasound session, when sonographers describe the placenta as baby's first home and a little sleeping bag.

The placenta mediates and also separates the mother and the fetus, making "their co-existence possible, by neutralizing their immunological reactions" (Santoro 2011: 76). It is both matter and meaning. A 1987 midwifery textbook aimed at Danish pregnant women and midwives notes,

> Even though the mother cake looks like a piece of raw liver, it has been the Lifetree for your child. You may want to take a closer look and see the difference between the rough part, which is turned towards the uterine wall, and the smooth part turned towards the child, which is like a soft velvet pillow, and study the network of blood vessels that has enabled your child to live and flourish inside your body. (Kitzinger 1979 212)

The placenta enacts cultural as well as kin significance. When buried underneath a tree, it becomes a generation builder, a symbol of genetic relatedness, or, in the case of lotus births, remains attached to the newborn. In the latter case, the placenta turns into a health resource and protector, or as noted by one of the interviewees, her daughter's "little red handbag" (figures 4.1–4.3).

Once expelled from the birthing body, the placenta becomes matter in need of a new place (Douglas [1966] 1984). Santoro theorizes that the placenta is *liminal tissue* "whose function is to connect, to mediate, embody contending versions of the political and societal bond" (Santoro 2011: 77), linking children with particular communities, rooting them in particular places as shown in the decision to bury the placenta underneath a tree (figures 4.2 and 4.3). When circulated as raw material into the pharmaceutical or cosmetic industry, however, the placenta moves into new biopolitical regimes (Santoro 2011). In this chapter, I use feminist cultural analysis (outlined in chapter 1) to develop these themes in more depth, conceptualized in this chapter in four analytical incisions. In the first analytical incision, the placenta is seen as biomedical evidence and reproductive waste. In the second analytical incision, I turn to the view of the placenta as consumable nutrients, re-naturalized as maternal love, while in the third analytical incision, I discuss the ways that the placenta is positioned as a rejuvenating ingredient in the development

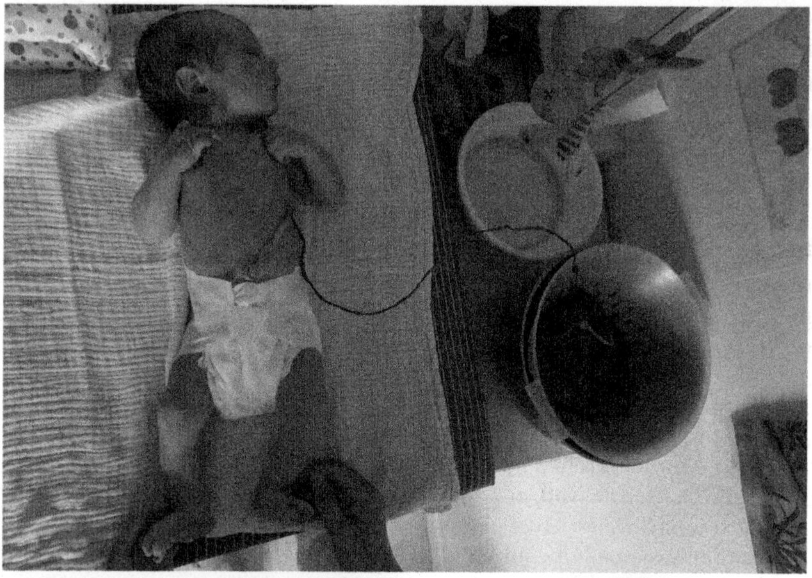

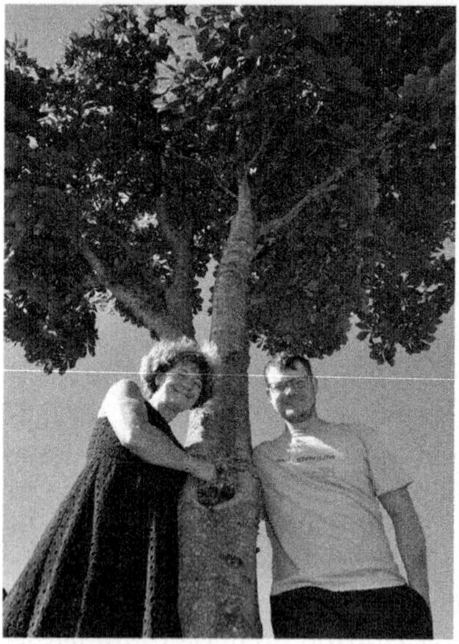

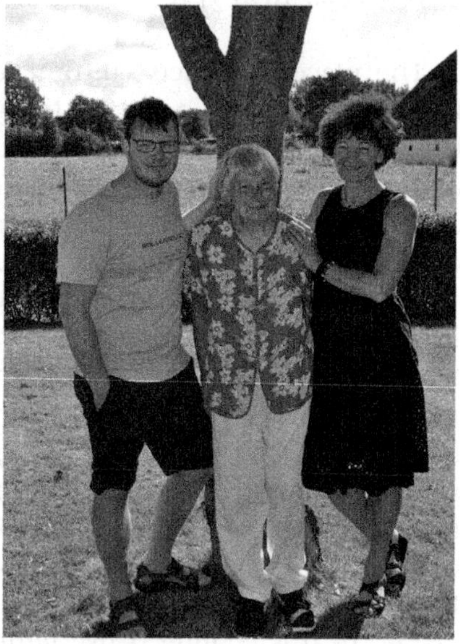

FIGURES 4.1, 4.2, and 4.3. Whereas the first photo represents a lotus birth in which the baby is not separated from the umbilical cord and the placenta until they separate on their own, figures 4.2–4.3 show a mother and son united by the tree planted and fertilized with the son's placenta. The mother also has a tree fertilized with her placenta planted in this family garden (the grandmother is present in the third photo), and two other sons have fruit trees planted in the same yard. Photos were taken and shared by the mother and reprinted with permission from all. The lotus birth photo was taken by the Danish family and reprinted with their permission.

of Japanese anti-aging and whitening creams and placenta shampoos. In the fourth and final incision, I discuss how placentas reemerge as bioart and, within the context of stem cell banking, turn into a form of responsible investment in family health.

Analytical Incision 1: Placentas as Biomedical Evidence and Reproductive Waste

In the Danish clinical practices, the placenta becomes biomedical evidence as well as biohazard waste. To the midwives working in the Danish public birthing clinics, the placenta is medical evidence, a biomedical indicator of the newborn baby's and mother's health and the woman's lifestyle during pregnancy. Conceptualized now as "afterbirth," the placenta becomes the focus of routinized clinical practices aimed at securing the health of the new mother as well as that of the newborn. Upon exiting the body, the placenta is weighed by the midwife, who also examines the appearance and feel of it. The midwife ensures that the placenta is intact (checking that no part of the placenta or the membranes have been left inside the uterus) and examines the umbilical cord to ensure that it has two arteries and one vein (Palmer 2015). She documents any abnormalities, such as a thin placenta, which may be a sign of smoking or maternal high blood pressure, indicating a less than optimal environment for the baby's growth.[11] In the case of abnormalities, or in cases of preterm babies or birth defects, the placenta is sent out for further testing. In these enactments, the placenta achieves biomedical agency: it reflects or "gossips" on the pregnant woman's lifestyle. For example, gray calcified areas in the placenta reveal smoking during pregnancy, leading to questions about fetal health as well as "good" or proper maternal behavior during pregnancy.

In clinical practice, the placenta is admired as a "life generator," examined as "biomedical evidence," and discarded as "waste." Expressing admiration when touching the fresh and warm placenta, the midwives sometimes display it to the new parents and encourage them to photograph it. In the public clinic, its status as afterbirth turns into reproductive waste, when, following the initial health checks, it moves from the midwife to the scale and into the yellow bag signaling biomedical refuse. Temperature plays a role as well. One midwife notes how her admiration of the placenta is disrupted and disturbed once it has turned into cold matter. Once cold, the placenta becomes biomedical waste en route to the incinerator. The fact that the placenta goes into a container with other tissue parts, as well as severed limbs, furthermore, cements its new status as abject (Kristeva 1982) and reproductive waste.

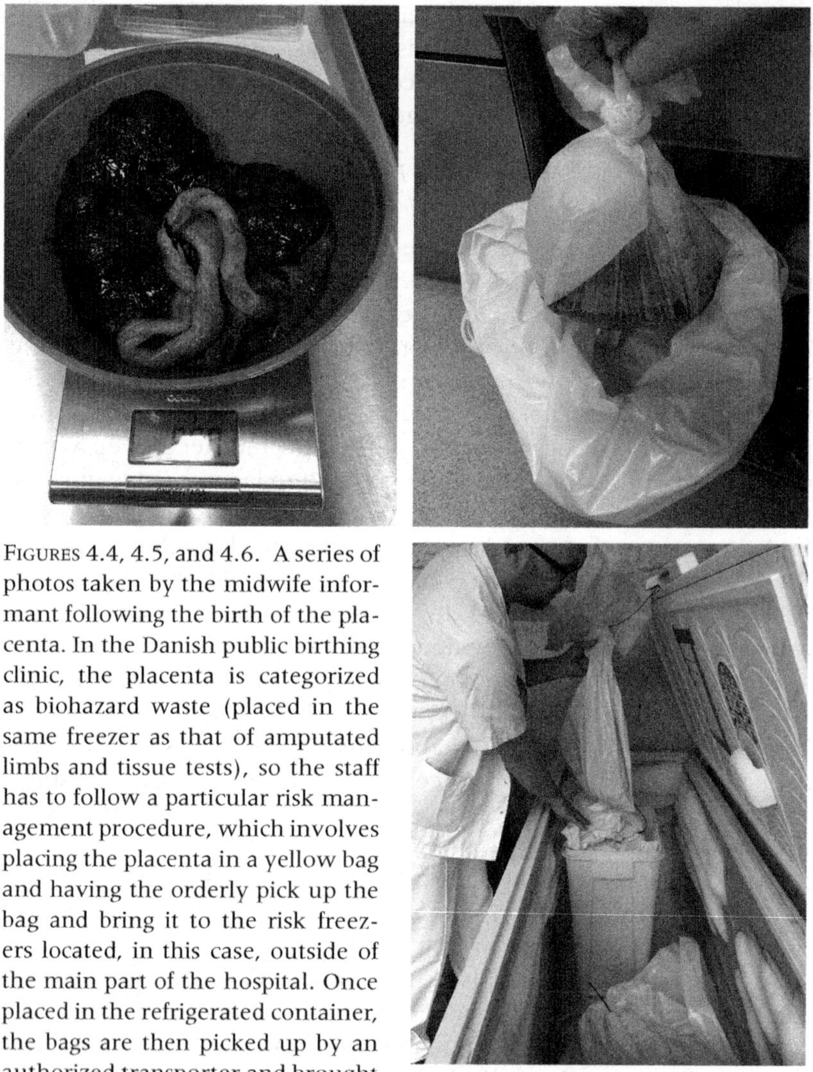

FIGURES 4.4, 4.5, and 4.6. A series of photos taken by the midwife informant following the birth of the placenta. In the Danish public birthing clinic, the placenta is categorized as biohazard waste (placed in the same freezer as that of amputated limbs and tissue tests), so the staff has to follow a particular risk management procedure, which involves placing the placenta in a yellow bag and having the orderly pick up the bag and bring it to the risk freezers located, in this case, outside of the main part of the hospital. Once placed in the refrigerated container, the bags are then picked up by an authorized transporter and brought to an incinerator. In the first photo (figure 4.4), the placenta is weighed and then transferred into a yellow bag to signal biohazard waste (figure 4.5). In figure 4.6, the orderly brings the bagged placenta to the waste container and presses it into another yellow container within it. All photos are reprinted with the permission of the midwife.

In the public clinical practices, the placenta loses its significance to the body that it came from when it is removed from the woman who has just given birth. The view of the placenta as waste is echoed in televised documentaries, as well as in social media responses to women who consume their own placentas. In the televised documentaries, the audience is warned of "potentially upsetting images," while in the 2015 Danish TV program on "perfect mothers," the placenta never leaves its reproductive past behind. Here, an acclaimed (male) chef prepares and tastes what is portrayed as a gourmet placenta meal and notes, "I still think it tastes of the birthing ward."[12] The positioning of the placenta as reproductive waste is echoed by the fact that, once it is expelled from the body, the placenta may mix with other bodily fluids, reinforcing the view of it as polluted matter. One obstetrician-gynecologist notes, "When you deliver, there are a lot of body fluids close together. You might have a bowel movement and it might touch the placenta. We can't promise it's not contaminated" (Pelley 2016).

However, its new status as reproductive waste is integral to the placenta's recirculation into (more) profitable contexts. As noted in chapter 1, placentas move from personal reproductive waste to profitable matter, recycled within "the infrastructures of capitalism and commodity culture" (Waldby and Cooper 2008: 83). The category of "waste" is consequently, as noted in chapter 1, a technical one. It legitimizes recirculation and enables other categories to emerge. When situated within the category of waste, the placenta is potential revenue-generating matter. One 33-year-old Danish farmer echoes this point when he notes his decision to collect, freeze, and redistribute porcine afterbirth. For him it is a welcome waste optimization procedure, generating a little over US$2 an afterbirth kilo, approximately US$15,000 a year: "I hang bags by the pigs. Every time we walk around, we wear a glove because the afterbirth has to be picked up as early as possible. Then, they are brought to the freezer" (Mikkelsen 2015). In this case, waste management is entangled with concrete practices (being present when the afterbirth arrives, wearing gloves, having bags ready, having a freezer large enough to contain afterbirth).

Bodily waste is not value-neutral (Kroløkke et al. 2016). This is also true in the case of the placenta. In the public clinical practices, the placenta is physically placed out of view (in the yellow bag, the refrigerated container). What Douglas ([1966] 1984) referred to as a search for purity is disrupted once placentas defy the regime of waste and enter other value regimes, such as those involving cooking and consumption. As waste-in-the-making, the placenta as food is debated and negotiated by preparers and consumers alike. In these constructions, the fact that the placenta is expelled from the inside of the body makes it an abject (Kristeva 1982). In the aforementioned Danish TV program, we learn that placenta is on the menu when the female TV host (dressed in fashionable Danish clothes and holding a fresh-looking placenta in her hands) notes that "mother's cake" will be served along with coffee. Questioning the appropriateness of placenta consumption and prior to tasting the delicious-looking placenta meal, she asks the chef, "Do you think it is disgusting that we are going to eat Maja's placenta? I am totally ambivalent about it. Yes and no. It is not from an animal, this thing. It is from a living human being. It is from a woman in Jutland" (the chef laughs). The ambivalence of eating what used to be a reproductive organ is pronounced, yet when combined with the fact that this placenta stems from a woman in Jutland (a regional area in western Denmark that is frequently stigmatized as being more rural), placenta consumption may even appear healthy and closer to nature. To Kristeva, however, the border between consumption and bodily expulsion is exactly what makes the placenta potentially repugnant: "It is thus not lack of cleanliness or health that causes abjection but what disturbs identity, system, order" (Kristeva 1982: 4). Similarly, the program host positions the placenta as similar to other forms of bodily expulsions: "It is something that is expelled from the body like a tear, a nail or a bugger."

This analytical incision has highlighted how the placenta, expelled from the inside of the body, is managed primarily as biomedical waste within the Danish public clinical setting. This is also illustrated in the interview study of supporters and also non-supporters of placenta consumption, when Dickinson et al. (2017) use the rhetoric of disgust and grotesqueness to delineate how non-supporters see eating one's own organ as a form of animality through the juxtaposition of two incompatible things (eating and human organ). Similarly, Gelis notes that the placenta exists in the twilight zones of birth: "produced by the body, and from its depths, the placenta is in the twilight zone of childbirth" (Gelis 1991: 165). In the quest to manage the placenta as an organ that once resided inside the uterus to now being discharged from it (Douglas [1966] 1984), it becomes troubled reproductive matter—best relegated as abject and waste, or as noted by one non-supporter in the Dickinson et al. study, "What if your own toe fell off, would you eat it?" (Dickinson et al. 2017: 11). Having discussed the ways that placentas in clinical practices, as well as in televised documentaries and in interviewee accounts, move from being seen as a vital reproductive organ to biomedical evidence to troubled waste, I turn to a more detailed analysis of placentas as consumable matter.

Analytical Incision 2: Nature's Bloody Mary[13] *and Motherly Love*

In a BBC4 cooking show TV Dinners, two women are busy turning a large, bloody (red) placenta into brown garlic pâté served on small slices of bread to approximately twenty guests, while the male voiceover comments: "I'll warn you now. If you don't like watching people eat bits and pieces of meat that has come out of their vagina, look away."[14] Women who choose to eat their placenta (placentophagia) reimagine the placenta as being separate from waste and cannibalism.[15] In this analytical incision, I first discuss how eating the placenta transitions from an act of eating one's own organs to becoming an act of motherly love. The placenta moves from having no ontological value to an act of gender empowerment, distributed back to the woman that it came from: *It's your own iron, so you can absorb it* (Maxted 2014). It becomes a new form of biological property, or as noted by Waldby and Mitchell in reference to cord blood, "The private cord blood account creates a legal relationship between person and tissue fragment that negotiates some of the aporias opened up by the contemporary tissue economies" (Waldby and Mitchell 2006: 123). I will return to this discussion of the placenta as a bioasset in my fourth analytical incision and in the conclusion to this book, but now simply note that the transformation of the placenta into a consumable item[16] turns placenta consumption into a form of responsible mothering.

When situated in the nexus between reproductive waste and human organ, placenta consumption becomes a repulsive act resembling a form of cannibalism. Goldblatt situates the eating of human organs as the ultimate taboo, "repugnant at best, criminal and blasphemous at worst" (Goldblatt 2000: 477). The theme of cannibalism can be found in various literary works and historical accounts: from the myth of Saturn, who ate his own children, to the suspense novels of Thomas Harris, which were later made into films, featuring Dr. Hannibal (the cannibal) Lecter, played by Anthony Hopkins, who enjoyed human flesh along with a bottle of Italian Chianti. Frequently surrounded with mysticism and revolt, and positioned in close proximity to savage cultures, cannibalism also becomes a means to survive, as evidenced in the stories of the Donner party, who in 1846 resorted to cannibalism, and the 1972 Andean plane crash, in which the survivors similarly consumed their dead fellow passengers (Goldblatt 2000). Cannibalism as a theme reappeared in the early 2000s, when a forty-two-year-old German man was arrested for killing and eating a young man, who had agreed to die and be eaten. Once again, the cannibalistic act was repositioned into a gourmet meal when the accused recounted consuming the now fried, garlicky flesh with, in this case, a bottle of South African red wine.[17] In fact, Gelis argues that the image of women eating their placenta may conjure up cultural imaginations of devouring human flesh, perhaps even transgressing gendered behaviors in eating human children: "The lurking image of the mother eating her placenta perhaps concealed another lurking image: the mother devouring her own children" (Gelis 1991: 166).

But whom or what are these women eating? Part them or part baby? In the placenta consumers' account, the placenta is repositioned as neither. In contrast, placenta consumption becomes an act of gender empowerment (see also Dickinson et al. 2017; Kroløkke et al. 2016). On its website, the British organization Independent Placenta Encapsulation Network (IPEN) features four women—all smiling—who situate placenta encapsulation as an international women's health issue (the United Kingdom, Ireland, Spain, Hong Kong, Australia, Japan, and Singapore are mentioned) as well as a fundamental challenge to Western birthing practices in the slogan: "Bringing the placenta back into post-birth healing since 2009."[18] As noted by one of the IPEN supporters, and in reference to her choice to consume the placenta combined with the recent EU ruling against third-party encapsulation,[19] "How can men in suits take that away? Women shouldn't be told they can't do something during their own birth. She has the right to do whatever she wants" (Kelly 2014), comparing the decision to have a trained encapsulation provider assist in the process with "a woman's right to choose where she would like to give birth" (Lynnea 2015). Equating placenta consumption with choice, IPEN features a photo on their website with a woman holding a sign saying, "My Placenta. My Choice."[20] Consuming one's placenta becomes situated as a newfound freedom or as a form of taking back women's own body parts. In this positioning, placenta consumption becomes a form of women's "human rights" (Lynnea 2015), liberating women from oppressive Western birthing practices, acknowledging and valuing women's bodies while simultaneously positioning them within recognizable metaphors of Western individualism (control, autonomy, and personal output) (Dickinson et al. 2017; Franklin et al. 2000; Kroløkke et al. 2016).

In the IPEN marketing information, as well as in interviewee accounts, the decision to turn the placenta into nutritional material is situated in close proximity to ancient, natural, Eastern practices. Drawing upon a back-to-nature argument, one mother says, "I love eating everything that comes from nature, and the placenta is some of the most natural. I would rather drink a smoothie with placenta in the morning than a cup of coffee" (Kjær 2013). Similarly, the London Placenta Centre positions placenta consumption as a long-lost, ancient (natural) practice: "The placenta can further continue its nourishing role as a nutritional supplement beyond the womb and in China, placenta has been used in natural healing and nutrition for thousands of years."[21] In this narrative, placenta consumption becomes instinctual, as noted in Lisa's interviewee account: "It makes sense and contains hormones and nutrients, and what a waste to just toss it out. It makes sense other animals do it, there is a reason for that."

Albeit positioned as a form of pure nature (Dickinson et al. 2017), placenta consumption is managed in a particular way. Images of mammals tearing and eating their placentas are replaced with an image of a delicious-looking smoothie or a pill—packaged and presented in a distinctly feminized form (figures 4.7–4.8.). The

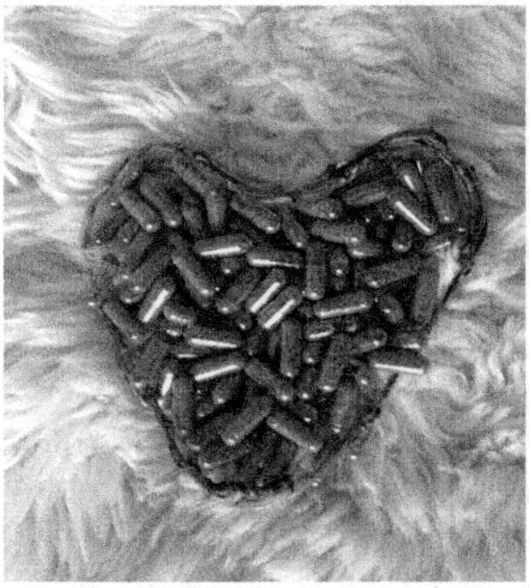

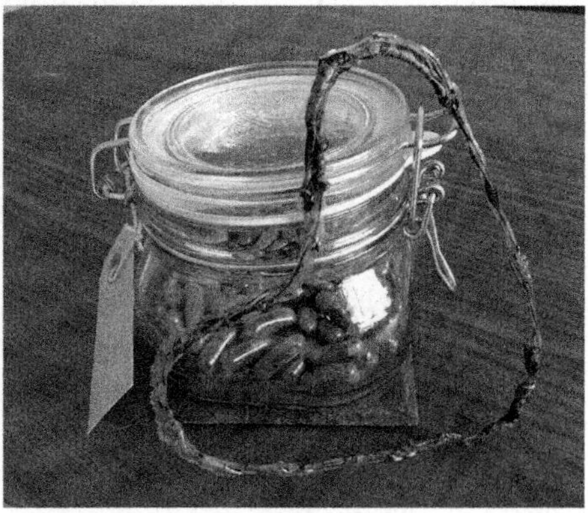

FIGURES 4.7 and 4.8. Placenta encapsulation and dried umbilical cord. While placenta encapsulation can be done by women themselves, when performed by a trained placenta specialist in Denmark, it costs approximately US$140, including pickup of the placenta and delivery of the placenta capsules. A similar service in London (including pickup and drop-off) performed by the London Placenta Centre costs between 220 British pounds (US$300) (for encapsulation) to 50 British pounds (US$66) for a raw placenta smoothie.[22] Photos are taken by one Danish interview participant and reprinted with her permission.

animality of placenta consumption is aesthetically and also rhetorically managed and restored within a gendered understanding of appropriate consumption (Kroløkke et al. 2016). In the image of the placenta as a vitamin or a pill, the placenta is repackaged and reconstituted as clean and pure matter, transformed through slow cooking and the use of a blender into a healthy snack or an empowered "vitamin Me."

Placenta consumption is not merely about nutrition, however. It gets re-entangled with the personal relations that produced it. Throughout the interviews and also in the mediated accounts on placenta consumption, the placenta is closely affiliated with maternal love, positioned, in this script, as more akin to the heart than its actual position (and appearance and also taste) near the liver. The notion of the placenta as an entanglement of love and affection, in the making of the baby as a love object, is reiterated in figures 4.7 and 4.8, where the umbilical cord reappears in the shape of a heart and placenta-encapsulated pills are placed inside it. Similarly, Tine in her interview situates the placenta as a sign of her already existing love for this baby, yet she also engages a particular heteronormative temporality involving "all those changes in life, from getting your menstruation, getting married, having a child, dying and having to give birth." As an affective bioobject, the placenta is no longer merely edible. Rather, it becomes a symbol of a maternal love object, naturalizing affects of love as inherently belonging to the mother-child relationship.

The interviews show that consuming one's own placenta is strongly motivated by a fear of postpartum depression, loss of energy, and potential lack of breast milk; thus, in some ways, placenta consumption is motivated by a desire to perform "good" mothering. As noted by one woman who had three placenta smoothies and encapsulated the remaining placenta, "I have had energy. I bonded with this baby. Everything is so much better. I got a little teary when my milk came in but that was the only mental wobble. I had the baby on a Thursday, and three days later I was cooking the Sunday dinner. I've been on the trampoline with my toddler" (Maxted 2014). To this extent, placenta consumption enables a new mother to fulfill a type of intensive mothering (Hays 1996; Kroløkke et al. 2016), allowing her to continue the routine of taking care of a newborn while also nurturing other children, managing the household, and maintaining a positive outlook on life ("that was the only mental wobble"). As noted in this analytical incision, placenta consumption discursively as well as affectively draws on the idea of maternity as a neoliberal project in which new mothers bear the responsibility for their own individual well-being, as well as that of their babies, extended to and echoed in the testimony of the aforementioned grandmother making her daughter a placenta smoothie: "I feel a bit like Martha Stewart."[23]

Analytical Incision 3:
Placentas as an Anti-aging and Whitening Commodity

The placenta engages in another layer of mobility, when it moves from the individual woman (an unprofitable context) to the profitable contexts of the cosmetic industry. In this case, biomedical matter is redistributed from one woman (where it came from) to other (mostly) women. It becomes a sellable ingredient, now remade into lotions or shampoos and promising the upward mobility associated with white, ageless, spotless skin and bouncy, straight, shiny hair. In this framing, the placenta gains industrial and commercial value, for example when it is returned to "nature" in the promise of "naturally" white and blemish-free skin (Kroløkke et al. 2016). In this analytical incision, I discuss how the placenta emerges as a vital ingredient in whiteness and youth-generating commodities.

During the 1950s and 1960s, the placenta became an ingredient in mass-marketed cosmetic products to be consumed by bourgeois, European women. In a lecture delivered to the Society of Cosmetic Chemists, Myddleton stresses about the use of placenta extracts that the "very definite effects on the rejuvenation and general toning of the human skin have been described after external application of cosmetic preparations containing these extracts" (Myddleton 1959: 202). The understanding of the placenta as an anti-aging material was echoed in European cosmetics commercials at the time. For example, in an old newspaper ad for the German cosmetic company Hormocenta (available during the 1950s), the placenta's beautifying and youthful qualities are extolled through the images of a white woman and a male scientist (featured in the lower left-hand corner of the ad). This message is similarly present in Helena Rubinstein's "Tree of Life" ad during the 1950s, where placenta-based lotion is equated with the production of the presumably soft skin of a white, attractive model whose face rests against the soft skin of a nude white baby. Here the placenta becomes a reinvention of nature visually depicted in the interface of the nude white skin of the baby and the woman's white skin.[24]

The modern European woman could now modify her skin tone as she pleased. She could not only become whiter and wrinkle-free, diminishing the aging spots on her skin, but she could also gain access to a liberated future through the mechanisms of individual self-control (Hunter 2011). In fact, Hunter situates whiteness products within modernity, noting that "the connection between modernity and body manipulation is distinctive from the centuries-old trend of 'decorating or ornamenting' the body, and is really about reshaping the body to present a new body as 'natural'" (Hunter 2011: 146). Similarly, in the Japanese commercials, placenta cosmetics enable women to get in touch with their long-lost nature (Kroløkke et al. 2016). As noted by Kroløkke et al., "The placenta moves from its life-giving potentiality and recycles to re-vitalize old (dead) skin" (Kroløkke et al. 2016: 10). This is also vital to the Japanese market for cosmetics in which skin-care products with a multipurpose appeal are generally seen as more attractive products.[25]

The case of Japan is especially interesting. Not only is Japan one of the world's leading national markets in cosmetics, with US$13 billion sales in 2016, but their marketing materials have been suc-

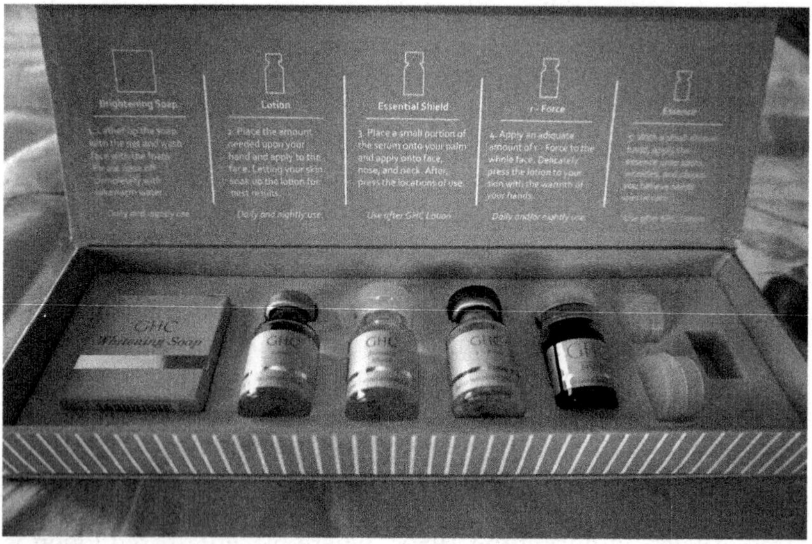

FIGURE 4.9. This image reveals a small trial package of various human placenta–based cosmetic products given to me by Japan Bio Products on my visit to the headquarters in Tokyo. The package consists of brightening soap (written as whitening soap), lotion, essence, essential shield, r-force, and a special concentrate aimed at deep wrinkles. If bought in the United States, the GHC Human Placenta skincare line costs approximately US$150, while the porcine-based GHC ultimate AA cosmetics line run US$144.[26] Photo taken by author.

cessful in employing a "Zen" and "a face from the East" image primarily to the regional Asian market including, China and Singapore (Umemura and Slater 2017: 890). As noted by Umemura and Slater (2017) in their genealogy and discussion of the Japanese cosmetics company Shiseido, the Asian consumer's imaginary of Japan as "cool" helped Shiseido establish a strong presence in the Chinese market, for example. Meanwhile, the Japanese citizen spends more money per year on cosmetics than any other consumer, averaging US$223 per capita per year, compared to US$139 in the United States and US$171 in France.[27] Some of the most viable Japanese products include anti-aging, skin-lightening, and moisturizing cosmetics.

In the Japanese cosmetic industry, a preference for whiteness and Japanese origin is embedded in the choice of "carefully selected" Japanese-made placenta extract or in the claim of the product being "100% Japanese."[28] Beauty becomes a form of social capital (Hunter 2005), and the currently dull and wrinkled skin is transformed and turned into soft and "natural" baby skin (Kroløkke et al. 2016: 11). The commercials combine racial understandings of whiteness as capital with nationalized understandings of superior hygiene and quality, as exemplified in the decision to use placentas from Japan and Denmark. In a case involving porcine placentas, the Japanese cosmetic company Hirosophy uses Danish pig afterbirth in its "Cell Bright series" products, promising the latest skin science technology combined with the highest quality *divine* placenta, assisting women of all age groups to engage in this rediscovery of smooth skin.[29] In this manner, whiteness, nationality, and origin (Japan and Denmark) are combined in the production and promise of "quality products," crossing over human/animal borders in the production of cosmetic products made out of Danish pigs' afterbirth matter, meanwhile reiterating particular geopolitical regions (such as Northern Europe) as not only safe(r) (with good hygiene and quality life) but attractive.

The promised transformation embedded in placenta cosmetics, however, extends beyond the immediate goal of whiter, younger facial features. In other words, placenta-based cosmetics are not merely about "yearning for whiteness" (Glenn 2008). The market in whiteness engages the promise of racial upward mobility and combines the ability to enjoy the racial privileges associated with whiteness with different forms of capital: "Light skin tone can be transformed into social capital (social networks), symbolic capital (esteem or status), or even economic capital (high-paying job or promotion) (Hunter 2011: 145). When situated within the nexus of skin color stratification and racist ideologies (Hunter 2002, 2005, 2007, 2011), whiteness upholds the promise of a better future, and here placenta-based products turn into rightful forms of individual self-enhancement. As noted on Japan Bio Products' US website, "Free your skin of impurities with GHC Soap HP for a silky, clear shine."[30] Glenn echoes this when she notes that the preference for lighter skin is not merely about whiteness but symbolic capital that improves one's ability to "free oneself," thereby becoming a "good catch" and holding out the promise of being a good reproductive body, reproducing intergenerational and reproductive upward mobility "in the production of light-skinned children" (Glenn 2008: 282).

Whereas Hunter (2005, 2011) discusses whiteness within the context of the African American and Mexican American communities in the United States, Glenn (2008) surveys the link between skin-bleaching and colonialism, and Arudou discusses the racial capital of whiteness in the Japanese context, which is particularly pertinent in the making of cosmetic products: "Japan's upper classes and historical figures are generally framed with very pale skin, while Japanese women, seen mostly indoors, are generally rendered whiter than men" (Arudou 2013: 49). In the case of Japanese placenta-based cosmetics, skin tone intersects with both class and nationality. Whiteness becomes a marker of being upper class—even Japanese nationality—framing darker-skinned persons as "lower class" or "foreigners" (Arudou 2013). As a marker of class and wealth, white skin gets equated with wealth, aristocracy, and power in the Japanese context (Glenn 2008). In fact, Glenn (2008) positions the Japanese market in cosmetic products as deeply embedded within a desire for whiteness, reiterated in the choice to use "white," or connotations associated with "whiteness," in product names such as the "Cell *Bright* Series" (Hirosophy) and "*White* Label" (Miccosmo). In this manner, placenta-based cosmetic products are reimagined as pure (white) and ageless nature (Kroløkke et al. 2016).

In the material, the placenta is de-personalized and re-personalized along gendered, racial, and national lines. The president of the Japanese cosmetic company Hirosophy features a photo of herself on the company website, displaying a pale, blemish-free, and wrinkle-free face, along with a list of placenta products, all made for her and tested by her. This company exclusively uses the afterbirth from Danish organic pigs, we learn.[31] The choice to use Danish porcine placentas has been made in part due to the Danish rules and regulations, while, as already noted, it draws upon the idea of Danish quality:

> Most Japanese pigs are vaccinated in order to prevent their developing infections from eating imported fodder from foreign countries; some of the vaccinations are mixed with antibiotics. We regard the safety of Japanese pigs not to be completely guaranteed. Danish pigs are grown under consistent national guidelines, including the distribution of the fodder for pigs. About 80% of the fodder is Danish made and all the contents are strictly regulated.

The company concludes that Danish pigs might be "healthier than humans living in the modern big cities,"[32] making a reference to the overcrowded, large Japanese cities and drawing on an understanding of Scandinavian health, hygiene, clean air, and overall quality. Nevertheless, the company's stamp of "Made in Japan," on all of its products is an attempt to signify superior quality and safety.

The re-personalized nature of the placenta's beautifying potential is similarly present, albeit in a completely different set of empirical material, when the founder and director of IPEN recounts her placenta's redeeming qualities in keeping her skin moist and her hair attractive: "And my skin and hair . . . oh, I felt like a supermodel! Beyoncé and Jennifer Lopez don't smother their faces in expensive deer placenta face cream for no reason" (Schrief 2015). While the director uses Beyoncé and Lopez as celebrity examples of placenta consumption, these two entertainers are interesting in other ways as well. Beyoncé and Lopez have both negotiated race and sexuality in the production of their successful careers (Bernardi 2008), and they have become exemplars of what Hunter (2007) calls forms of colorism, in which lighter-skinned African Americans and Latinas in the United States have become more successful and palatable to a white audience than their darker-skinned performers. Similarly, in the promotion of their text *Skin Deep: How Race and Complexion Matter in the "Color-Blind" Era,* Herring et al. (2003) ask: Why did Michael Jackson become lighter as he became more successful and O.J. Simpson darker as he was accused of murder? La Bella—a Minnesota-based company—is another case in point, as they intertwine placenta extract with race and class in the production of their placenta shampoo and conditioning.[33] La Bella promises its Hispanic female consumers "the secret to Latin Beauty," redefined through the use of human placenta extract, repackaged as shampoo and conditioner that produces distinctly straight, silky, shiny, long dark hair, and which is made to appear readily available on Amazon and in large chain stores such as Walmart and Target.[34]

This analytical incision has demonstrated that the placenta gains commercial value as beauty capital, engaging the promise of upward mobility yet also becoming a technology of self-empowerment, re-naturalized in the commercials and visual representations. As noted by Japan Bio Products, the placenta-derived lotion "normalizes skin regeneration" and works by (naturally) balancing women's hormones. In this incision, beautiful skin is equated to healthy skin—"Beautiful skin is healthy skin, and GHC human placenta cosmetics contain specific nutrients to support your specific needs"[35]—and thus, the company secures a multipurpose product of both beauty and health. Transformed into brightening and anti-aging lotion or creamy conditioner and shampoo (in the production of straight hair), placenta-based products testify to what Glenn positions as "white is right" (Glenn 2008: 298). The circulation of placentas into the cosmetic industry has generated its share of criticisms from unwilling providers, however. When a British hospital in Dorset reportedly provided placentas donated by British women, not to the expected medical research facilities but to the cosmetic industry, it created quite a media stir. One of the placenta providers commented, "I feel violated by what I have been through. It feels like they stole it because it was all done on false pretense. It's from my body. It's my DNA and I feel like they tricked it from me" (Sawer 2008). Meanwhile, the use of placentas in cosmetic and shampoo products is resolved in the reconstitution of the placenta as a "natural" ingredient. Here, the notion of the placenta as property matter ("my DNA") in the wrong place ("I feel like they tricked it from me") is contrasted with the view of the placenta as "natural." Consequently, the placenta is not a secretive ingredient in the cosmetic industry but rather a reinvigorating and core ingredient, promising the upward mobility associated with youthful, attractive, modern, fertile, and white female bodies.

Analytical Incision 4: From Bioart to Biological Investment

Consistent with the view of placenta practices as postpartum reinventions, placentas take on other values when they become bio-art or when they are situated within the speculative and profitable contexts of the stem cell industry. Here, placentas become affective, promissory, and also speculative investments.

As noted by one placenta service provider in the Portland, Oregon, area, placenta art puts the ART in PostpARTum.[36] Placenta prints are some of the more common art pieces, requiring only good paper and one fresh placenta. The artist wipes off excess blood, making the print using the remaining blood already covering the placenta. Placenta prints, available for around US$30, give the viewer a sense of the topography of the placenta, noting placenta "branches" and turning the placenta print into the recognizable "tree of life" image.[37] Line, a Danish woman who used her placenta to make placenta art, recollects standing alone after the birth in the middle of the night, "washing the placenta—she [the encapsulator] had asked me to do that. She had instructed me in what to do, and so I rolled out this ink, or whatever it is called, you know paint, on the mother cake." While Line was making placenta prints in the middle of the night, her boyfriend used the placental membrane to make a small drum: "That drum really meant a lot to him . . . and he was very concerned about where to hang it, because other people thought it was disgusting." The drum eventually hung in the kitchen window, available for public view, but its value remained mostly personal.

While placenta art resembles a form of birth and pregnancy memory management, romanticizing what could also be viewed as simply a large (bloody) organ, the placenta processed into a pill and consumed is a biological self-investment. One encapsulation service provider notes how the monstrosities of organ eating are avoided when the placenta is turned into "a jar of pills you can pop with your daily vitamins."[38] In this setup, the placenta vitamin infusion[39] enables the consumer to gradually reintroduce the nutrients lost during childbirth. Placenta consumption is constructed not only as being beneficial to the present-day health of the new mom but also as a method of delivering future curable assets. In her interview, Tine notes its potential as a medical treatment for her daughter and repeatedly refers to the placenta powder as "medicine": "I have frozen it in really small bags and have thought that if my daughter needs it, like if she gets a rash, then I will mix it with some oil and give it to her." The fact that the placenta can be converted from raw material to powder or pills makes it an even more mobile and compatible substance. Placenta encapsulation service providers chant while dehydrating and cooking the placenta at a low temperature for an extended period of time, grinding, packaging, and returning it into a medical-type form. The encapsulated pills can be taken daily or put in the freezer for later use. One placenta consumer says about the decision to save some of the placenta for later, "I am having the rest to make a placenta-infused vodka that is supposed to alleviate the symptoms of menopause" (Echlin 2011).

Here, the placenta engages in a transformation in value, becoming to the birthing woman a form of personal biological investment. As a form of own medicine, it turns into a personal "magic bullet" and an "energy booster" akin to other health supplements (Devlin 2014). The promise of health is clearly visible in the IPEN accounts, as well as in interviews with placenta consumers, when women recount escaping postpartum depression and feeling energetic quickly following the birth. The payoff here is a form of "biological self-enhancement" (Waldby and Mitchell 2006: 187), in which both the hopes for a happy maternity and also the susceptibility of health and energy loss following childbirth are linked. In a British documentary, following the birth of her grandchild, a birthing woman's mother quickly mixes bananas with large raw placenta chunks to help her daughter replace nutrients lost during birth (Smith 2015). The placenta gains nutritional value. While it once acted as a filter for the developing baby, it is now turned into a goldmine of vitamins that are crucial in helping the new mom with milk production and lowering the risks of postpartum depression, a testament to the placenta's role in the reproductive work during pregnancy and echoed in the fact that this woman's mother stresses that her daughter needs the placenta smoothie "ASAP."

When entangling with the private stem cell industry,[40] however, the placenta engages with a capitalist logic, defined by Rajan as a form of biocapitalism: "The articulation of a technoscientific regime, having to do with the life sciences and drug development, with an economic regime, overdetermined by the market" (Rajan 2007: 111). Cryopreserved at negative 196 degrees Celsius, whole placentas can be collected and stored at LifebankUSA, a biobank located in the United States, for the total price of US$3,500 (excluding the US$300 annual storage fee). Storing the placenta allows the company to collect stem cells from two prenatal sources of stem-cell-rich blood, increasing the potential number of stem cells available, offering "potential for new treatments in immune disorders, wound healing, organ transplant and growth." Placenta banking is a means to protect not only the child but also the family at large, including the mother herself ("You want the best for your baby and family. So do we").[41] In fact, acknowledging its unique relationship to the mother, Americord points to the importance of placenta storing for future maternal health: "This is a rare opportunity to bank on Mom! The outermost layer of the placenta contains mom's mesenchymal stem cells (MSCs). This means that mom can now store her own life-saving stem cells."[42] What is positioned as an intimate link between mother and child is reworked within biobanking into an investment in the family's and mother's health.

The private stem cell banks turn the *generative* capacities of the prenatal body into *regenerative* capacities (Waldby 2006a; 2006b).

According to Waldby, placental tissue becomes "biological venture capital" (Waldby 2006b: 63), reconstructed by LifebankUSA and also Americord into a form of intimate, private family property. Its value, however, is speculative as well as promissory. Nevertheless, placental blood turns into a private insurance that only some can afford. Similar to umbilical cord blood banking, biobanking promises to help parents avoid the uncertainty of available genetic material while also managing the risk of future illnesses with the development of new cutting-edge treatments (Ericson et al. 2000). When banking placenta tissue or cord blood, parents are banking a donation that is "exactly right for [*their*] child" (Ericsson et al. 2000: 64). In this construction of custom-made cures, placental tissue and blood are reframed into speculative, yet nevertheless intimate, investments. Banking not only serves as a source for curative materials, it also engages the affect of hope in the body's capacity for self-renewal. Brown et al. echo this when they use "'promissory' capital" as a discursive frame to understand cord blood banking, repositioning what has the appearance of abstract capital into doing "'the right thing' for a child's future" (Brown et al. 2006: 344).

Banking the placenta and placental blood is both speculative and promissory. Nevertheless, it is positioned as being a form of responsible parenting ("having more cells available may prove beneficial for new treatments in an emerging medical field").[43] As echoed by LifebankUSA, it provides not just *"more protection,* but *better protection."*[44] It is framed as new parents having to make an urgent choice, broken into three simple steps: collection, processing, and preservation. The clock on LifebankUSA's website stresses the medical urgency, reiterated by the word REMEMBER (written in pink and capitalized). An Asian American mom appears with her three children, including a newborn, to the right of the following text: "Stem cells from placenta tissue can only be collected and preserved right after a baby is born."[45] The highly urgent yet speculative nature of placenta banking is managed in light of the potential for future cures ("Banking the entire placenta offers potential for new treatments in immune disorders, wound healing, organ transplant and growth"),[46] as recorded in accounts of children having already been saved by these "family cells." For example, we learn about the story of a young boy named Quentin "whose sister's cord and placenta blood saved his life. Quentin entered remission after his transplant and was deemed cured of leukemia two years later."[47] Here, placenta and cord blood gain agency within the genetic kinship unit.

Imagined Placental Bodies

Placentas are interesting reproductive matter. Clearly, placentas circulate in vastly different practices, in and out of different repro-economies, and produce very different meanings. Conversations with Danish midwives reveal a history of placenta exchanges with the pharmaceutical industry in return for what the midwives called "placenta money,"[48] cash they use in the clinical practices toward a new departmental couch, a television set, or the departmental summer party. The placenta is reimagined as reproductive waste (unclean, expelled matter), a beauty agent (anti-aging and whitening ingredient) and promissory matter (a future cure) (Thompson 2005; Brown et al. 2006). In their critique of the stem cell industry, Brown et al. stress that the reimagination and subsequent redistribution of blood make biological matter promissory capital, linking what appears to be a personal service to a biological, industrial complex providing an "entry point into an increasingly private linkage between parenting and biomedicine" (Brown et al. 2006: 344). Similarly, as a raw resource, the placenta transcends inner and outer beauty when circulating into the cosmetic industry, packaged in select cosmetics and beautifying lines. For example, Hirosophy reinvents the placenta as a form of ideal production when the company promises the "highest amount of pure placenta extract," stressing its beauty and also its health promises.[49]

But what do these different enactments of placental waste and value do to our understanding of the reproductive body? In the construction of the placenta as a consumable entity, the reproductive body becomes both empowered and entrepreneurial: it becomes, as noted by Shail (2007) in his analysis of menstrual blood, a corporeal body. According to Shail, "The menstrual body following mass communication's re-materializing of the body produces and entails flows of waste that this economy *publicly* validates as the behavior not of the sexed body but of the corporeal" (Shail 2007: 93). Women consume their placentas to regain their strength, removing the placenta out of the realm of disgust and repositioning placenta consumption within the labor of love. The notion that "you are what you eat" is here redefined into a language of gender empowerment and a form of intensive mothering. However, this empowered and entrepreneurial placental reproductive body is managed in several ways. Notably, in using the classification of "novel food," the European Food and Safety Authority (EFSA) echoes an understanding of placenta consumption as potentially involving the consumption of hazardous waste. Defined as food that has not been consumed in the European Union before 1997, novel food seeking authorization within the EU has to undergo a scientific assessment to ensure its safety,[50] making the marketing of placenta products potentially illegal in the European Union:

> Under Regulation 258/97, a novel food or ingredient is defined as one that was not consumed to a significant degree in the European Community before 15 May 1997. Novel foods and food ingredients may only be marketed if they have been evaluated and authorized under the procedures defined in the regulation. Human placenta and products derived from human placenta have not been authorized under this regulation.[51]

The skeptical view of the placenta as a consumable item is similarly reiterated by the Danish food authorities, who, in a question about the use of placenta products, reposition the placenta as an inner organ and respond, "We have no prior evidence of the marketing of human inner organs as food."[52] Despite these potential legal barriers, placenta encapsulation services are flourishing online, making a long list of placenta-related products available (encapsulation, smoothies, homeopathic remedies, creams for mom and baby, as well as prints).

Throughout the empirical material, the understanding of the reproductive body as entrepreneurial interacts with an understanding of the reproductive body as a (neoliberal) regenerative ecosystem. In the practices involved in placenta consumption, as well as in the mediated accounts, what is good for the fetus is good for mom and, within the stem cell industry, also for everyone within the genetically related family unit. Here, individual self-responsibility ensures that women use placenta consumption as a means to fulfill their roles as intensive mothers (taking care of children, being energetic, maintaining a positive outlook on life, thinking about the family's future health, etc.). In this construction, the reproductive body is a purposeful body that redeems its own value through selective acts of preservation and consumption. This view is similarly present in the stem cell industry and in the case of biobanking. Here, the responsible parent takes care to preserve genetic material. It is now no longer simply a "vitamin Me" but, rather, a future cure and thus a family investment in health. In the latter case, the reproductive body becomes a speculative body, as well as a regenerative resource used to invest in the health of the nuclear family.

Throughout this material, the placental body is depicted as white, whether actually white or metaphorically producing white-like bodies, as is the case in the cosmetic industry in the production of whitening and anti-aging products. Whereas Japanese women are considered to be anonymous philanthropic bodies that willingly (and without any compensation) provide the Japanese pharmaceutical and cosmetic industry with placenta tissue, the bodies that reappear in the mediated accounts, including the marketing material of the Japanese cosmetic products and La Bella's shampoo commercials, constitute distinctly middle-class, white, slim, feminized, young, attractive bodies. While the placenta moves into the cosmetic industry as a vital ingredient, the product itself promises the production of desirable bodies. In this context, the placenta consumer engages her own upward mobility not only by becoming whiter and younger but also by gaining access to the privileges associated with reproductive, transformable, and mobile bodies.

From Waste to Speculative Assets

The starting point in this chapter was how the placenta moves from waste (to me) to waste in a more general sense (biohazard waste in the clinical practices), regenerative value (encapsulated pills), beauty capital (anti-aging cosmetics and shiny hair products), and biocapital (future cures and treatments). Clearly, the placenta has value in the double sense of the word: it achieves market value when exchanged, and it has value as personalized alternative health medicine when consumed by individual women, thereby accumulating personal and kinship value. Consequently, the placenta gains value in its movement through various institutions, involving very different practices. As noted by Frow, "Value is an effect of the circulation of objects *between* regimes of value" (Frow 2003: 35). From the birthing body to the scale, the midwife's examination, the yellow bag, the biohazard containers (where the placenta mixes with other tissue and limbs), and the incinerator, as well as the blender, the oven, the factory/corporation, and other consumers, the placenta enters different regimes of value.

Placentas become waste material in one context (managed by medical professionals, collected and transported to the incinerator) yet potential value in another (raw material—at times in need of processing). In this circulation, and notably in the management of it, placentas gain double promissory and speculative value. While, in the case of the cosmetic and anti-aging industry, placentas become revenue-generating as a raw material developed into commodities sold transnationally, the decision to encapsulate or eat the placenta engages a different process of valuation. Sympathetic to the idea that the bioeconomy must be understood not only with regard to processes of commodification but also as a process of "assetization" (Birch 2016: 9), I note that placentas gain value not merely as capitalized and tradable properties but also in and through their management and ritualization practices (when the encapsulation preparer chants while cleaning and processing the placenta, for example). When eaten or encapsulated, placentas are neither revenue-generating nor tradable, but they are in fact unique and impossible to replicate. In this context, they become gendered resources or assets with speculative own future health benefits.

Notes

The analysis in this chapter relies on previously published material in Dickinson, E., K. A. Foss, and C. Kroløkke. 2016. "Empowering Disgust: Redefining Alternative Postpartum Placenta Practices." *Women's Studies in Communication* 40(1): 111–28 and in Kroløkke, Dickinson, and Foss 2016, "The Placenta Economy. From Trashed to Treasured Bio-Products, *European Journal of Women's Studies*, iFirst: 1–15.

1. Because interview studies are exempt from IRB approval in Denmark, I have followed the guidelines stipulated by the European Science Foundation (ESF) on good research practice. This entails that informed consent, anonymity, and privacy have been given and all participants have been met with openness and integrity. For more information on the ESF guidelines see ALLEA—All European Academies, "The European Code of Conduct for Research Integrity, Revised Edition," European Commission, 2017, http://ec.europa.eu/research/participants/data/ref/h2020/other/hi/h2020-ethics_code-of-conduct_en.pdf (retrieved January 2018).
2. The project involved a total of thirty-five interview participants located in Denmark, the United States, as well as Australia, where one woman was located at the time of the interview.
3. I visited one placenta preparer in Denmark and interviewed two midwives that run their own private birthing clinic in a posh Copenhagen neighborhood, as well as three other midwives working in the Danish public birthing clinics. I also held ten informal conversations with midwives working in public clinics.
4. One midwife agreed to photograph the routine practices undertaken at the public clinic where she works. The rules and regulations surrounding placenta management are the same throughout the country, yet they are managed differently in the private clinics where placenta consumption is presented as an option to all the pregnant women.

5. The online search using the words "placenta," "eat," and "brit" generated 443,000 search results, while a similar search using the Danish words "moderkage" and "spis" generated a total of 1,040 results. The first ten pages were examined and included in the online archive.
6. The Danish farmer receives 15 DKK per kilo (approximately US$2), and when averaging 123 kilos a week, the extra annual income is close to 100,000 DKK (US$15,000) (Mikkelsen 2015).
7. In the Q&A section of Hirosophy's website, Danish pigs are situated as healthier than humans living in big cities: http://www.hirosophy.co.jp/en/qa/index.html (retrieved May 2015).
8. I interviewed members of the farm association in Denmark and talked with one Danish company that sends porcine placentas to Japan. In addition, I included the online marketing material of A LifebankUSA Advantage, based in the United States, which picks up and stores placenta tissue for own later use. The cost of preserving cord blood, placenta blood, and the placenta itself varies, but according to LifebankUSA, it is approximately US$3,500 plus an additional annual storage fee of US$300. For more information see: Health Grove, http://cord-blood-banks.healthgrove.com/l/16/LifebankUSA (retrieved October 2017).
9. According to the FDA, cosmetic products do not need approval to be marketed to consumers, yet companies must not mislead, and they have the legal responsibility that their products are safe for consumers. U.S. Food and Drug Administration, "Cosmetics Q&A: Why Are Cosmetics Not FDA Approved?," updated 22 February 2018, http://www.fda.gov/Cosmetics/ResourcesForYou/Consumers/ucm135709.htm (retrieved September 2016).
10. The European Commission's definition of "Novel Food" was updated 22 February 2018 and can be found at their website: http://ec.europa.eu/food/safety/novel_food_en (retrieved October 2016).
11. This information is based on interview with a midwife in June 2016.
12. *De perfekte mødre* (The perfect mothers), a Danish television program airing on Danish channel DR2, 5 December 2015.
13. This reference to placenta consumption in general and placenta smoothies in particular is made by Maxted (2014).
14. The BBC cooking show is titled "TV Dinners" (1998); clip is available on YouTube, https://www.youtube.com/watch?v=5OXSN3iVWB8 (retrieved October 2016).
15. According to the Independent Placenta Encapsulation Network (2014), an estimated four thousand British women practiced placentoghagy from 2009 to 2014 (Maxted 2014).
16. The most common form of placenta consumption is encapsulation. Following birth, the placenta is dehydrated and ground into a powder, encapsulated into pills that can then be eaten for weeks, or when put into the freezer, the powder can be consumed even later in life such as when the woman goes through menopause.

17. The case received considerable media attention in Germany as well as abroad. Armin Meiwes admitted to having cut off Bernd Jürgen Armando Brandes's penis, which they jointly then tried (yet failed) to eat. Meiwes subsequently stabbed Brandes to death and hung his body up to dry. During the following ten months, he consumed twenty kilograms of Brandes's flesh. He received, during the appeal trial, life imprisonment. For more information, see the Wikipedia article on Meiwes: https://en.wikipedia.org/wiki/Armin_Meiwes (retrieved April 2018).
18. IPEN, http://www.placentanetwork.com/ (retrieved August 2016). IPEN has now five instructors located in six different countries (on three continents) and offers placenta remedy training to women with previous training in pregnancy, birth, or post-natal support. While no formal requirements exist (such as formal midwifery education), IPEN mentions not only the safety of the prepared placenta supplements but also the risks associated with cross-contamination to the preparer.
19. While women can choose to encapsulate their own placentas in the European Union, the placenta's potential classification as a "novel food" has been debated. According to the European Union, a novel food is a food that does not have a history of being consumed prior to 1997. Consequently, companies offering "novel foods" to potential customers are restricted in regards to their marketing and what services they can provide until they go through a process of authorization. IPEN still awaits the EU novel food safety regulations final decisions, which are expected in late 2017. More information on the EU Food Standards Agency classification on novel food can be found at https://www.food.gov.uk/science/novel/faqs (retrieved October 2017).
20. This rhetoric is found on: IPEN, "My Placenta, My Choice," http://www.placentanetwork.com/my-placenta-my-choice/ (retrieved June, 2016).
21. London Placenta Centre, http://www.placentacentre.co.uk (retrieved September 2016).
22. For more information see London Placenta Centre booking form, http://www.placentacentre.co.uk/wp-content/uploads/2017/08/Booking-form_2017.pdf (retrieved October 2017).
23. Video of the management of a placenta and transformation into a post-partum placenta smoothie: Youtube, https://www.youtube.com/watch?v=szSsXpcYf6s (retrieved August 2016).
24. Several of the European ads on placenta lotions can be seen at Cosmetics and Skin, http://cosmeticsandskin.com/cdc/placenta.php (retrieved November 2017).
25. An executive summary of the cosmetics industry in Japan, carried out by the U.S. Department of Commerce in 2016, cements the country as one of the world's largest markets for cosmetics and personal care products.

26. For more information on pricing and availability, visit JBP USA, https://jbpglobalusa.com/collections/ghc-placental-extract-cosmetics-1/products/ghc-ultimate-aa-placental-cosmetics (retrieved October 2017).
27. The figures in this paragraph are provided by the Executive Summary of Personal Care and Cosmetics Products, Country Guide Japan, carried out by the U.S. Department of Commerce, 2016.
28. See the Miccosmo White Label, http://www.miccosmo.co.jp/english/wl.html (retrieved May 2016).
29. See Hirosophy products, http://www.hirosophy.co.jp/cn/ (retrieved August 2016).
30. See Japan Bio Products Co., Ltd., "Products: GHP Soap HP," http://jbpglobal.placenta.co.jp/product/ghc-soap-hp/ (retrieved October 2017).
31. For more information see: Hirosophy, http://www.hirosophy.co.jp/cn/ (retrieved May 2015).
32. For more information see: Hirosophy, http://www.hirosophy.co.jp/en/qa/index.html (retrieved May 2015).
33. For more information about the product visit La Bella, http://www.labellabeauty.com (retrieved September 2016).
34. La Bella products can be bought at several stores, which can easily be located on the La Bella website: http://labellabeauty.com/en/where-to-buy-2/?address=01002. Prices vary, yet two La Bella products (shampoo and conditioner, for example) run approximately US$15 for shampoo and conditioner.
35. JBP Global USA· GHC Human Placenta Skincare—with Free Shipping!," https://jbpglobalusa.com/products/ghc-human-placenta-skincare (retrieved October 2017).
36. Portland Placenta Services website, http://www.portlandplacentaservices.com/placenta-prints--keepsakes.html (retrieved September 2016).
37. A long list of placenta-oriented services, including the making of placenta prints, is available on the Portland Placenta Services website: http://www.portlandplacentaservices.com/placenta-prints--keepsakes.html (retrieved October 2017).
38. Natural Afterbirth website, http://www.naturalafterbirth.com/why-would-i-eat-that.html (retrieved August 2016).
39. Ibid.
40. Banking the placenta entails, in the case of Americordblood.com, a one-time payment of US$1,999 or a plan of US$80 per month for twenty-four months. Americord, "What Is Placenta Tissue?," https://www.americordblood.com/banking/placenta-tissue/ (retrieved February 2016).
41. LifebankUSA, "What Is Advanced Biobanking?," http://www.lifebankusa.com/advanced-biobanking/ (retrieved September 2016).
42. Americord, "What Is Placenta Tissue?"
43. LifebankUSA, "What Is Advanced Biobanking?"
44. Ibid.
45. Americord, "What Is Placenta Tissue?"

46. LifebankUSA, "Why Bank Placental Blood?," https://www.lifebankusa.com/placenta-cord-blood-bank/placenta-blood-banking/ (retrieved September 2016).
47. Ibid.
48. Unfortunately, none of the midwives remembered the actual financial compensation. They did remember how "placenta money" assisted in hosting a summer party, buying a new sofa etc.
49. For more information about the Hirosophy products, visit the company's website: http://www.hirosophy.co.jp/ (retrieved August 2016).
50. European Commission, "Questions and Answers: New Regulations on Novel Food," 16 November 2015, http://europa.eu/rapid/press-release_MEMO-15-5875_en.htm (retrieved September 2016).
51. Change.org, "Placenta Services in Europe Should NOT Be Stopped by Novel Food Regulation (EC) 258/97," https://www.change.org/p/food-standards-agency-placenta-services-in-europe-should-not-be-stopped-by-novel-food-regulation-ec-258-97 (retrieved September 2016).
52. Danish food authorities, email correspondence with author, January 2016.

Conclusion

> The sperm travels out in a special vessel, which ensures it is maintained at the appropriate conditions. We understand the importance of this part of the program and that it proceeds without any risk to the samples and as such work with specialty couriers with experience transporting these important samples. As such, your samples are accompanied at all times until they are delivered safely to the laboratory staff at our partner clinics. ("Egg Donations in Ireland" 2017: 7)

In this conclusion I turn to the feminist cultural politics of reproduction and raise the following questions: Why do some reproductive donations lead troubled lives while others swiftly move into a globalized economy in reproductive waste and value? And how can a feminist cultural politics of reusability and extensibility contribute to our understanding of globalized reproductive fluids? A key argument throughout this book has been that reproductive tissue and fluids travel not only in a literal way, as illustrated in the above quote, but also culturally and metaphorically. In the above quote, sperm cells—not eggs—appear mobile. The narrative closely resembles one of science fiction or space travel; transportation and packaging technologies come to constitute a "special vessel," which entangles with reproductive matter ("sperm") and affects such as empathy and trust ("we understand the importance" and "without any risk") to make the mobility of frozen sperm seem safe and within the confines of caring relations ("your samples are accompanied at all times"). In this conclusion I discuss how feminist cultural politics addresses the ways that reproductive fluids move and entangle with politics and globality.

To do so, I turn to "gray thinking" (Knudsen and Frederiksen 2015) and discuss what I position as gift markets. I also return to the mobility turn, presented in chapter 1, to discuss, literally as well as imaginatively and metaphorically, the ways that reproductive fluids move as globalized practices. To Knudsen and Frederiksen (2015), gray thinking promotes ambiguity. It becomes an analytical lens that disrupts, defines, and highlights paradoxes. In chapter 3, for instance, we saw how egg providing in Spain entered different gray zones, producing very different imagined reproductive bodies, from informational bodies to exotic, rightful bodies and entrepreneurial bodies. Meanwhile, observations in the Spanish fertility clinic showed that fertility travel was, at times, choreographed and managed in a decidedly black-and-white manner. Not only was the desire for a child re-naturalized in the clinical discourses, but the provider's willingness to "donate" was also positioned as part and parcel of an innate Spanish altruism and willingness to "give" others the chance of motherhood. And whereas the international fertility travelers coming to Barcelona for egg providing entered an impressive, very modern, state-of-the art steel clinic, egg providers (local Spanish or immigrant women) entered a smaller, less imposing but also more intimate clinic located within a two-minute walk of the main clinic. Moreover, the clinic diminished the opportunities for gray interactions when they scheduled egg retrievals during the mornings and embryo implantations in the afternoons. In this manner, the clinic ensured that providers and recipients did not meet; although, in the recipient narratives recounted in chapter 3, any Spanish woman present in the clinic was seen as a potential provider.

In this conclusion I additionally use the mobility paradigm to discuss the processes of gifting and marketization and what these categorizations do to the ways that urine, oocytes, and placentas circulate and are viewed and practiced as exchangeable and globalized fluids. In line with gray thinking, I consistently use the term *gift markets* to challenge what I see as the false (and unproductive) dichotomy between the gift economy and the market economy. Instead, I inquire into the ways that gifting and commodification make certain movements and reproductive bodies possible, as well as into the ways that reproductive fluids travel in and out of commodity states. As noted by Kopytoff, commodification is a cultural process: "Commodities must be not only produced materially as things, but also culturally marked as being a certain kind of thing" (Kopytoff 1986: 64). Consequently, in this conclusion I turn to a feminist cultural politics of reusability and extensibility and argue that feminist cultural politics on reproductive waste and value needs to look beyond *what* is exchanged to *the acts* through which certain parts become exchangeable and enter different commodity states (Malmqvist 2012).

Mobility in the Gray Zones of Gift Markets

What is the relationship between reproductive donations and the gift market logics? As noted by Strathern, the gift/commodity tension makes the different relations between "persons," "things," "subjects," and "objects" visible (Strathern 1988: 19, 143). Moreover, and as evidenced in the three case chapters, the gift/commodity tension operates as a rhetorical framework, producing very different reproductive provider bodies. Whereas the philanthropic body relies heavily upon an altruism and gift-giving logic, the entrepreneurial body is strongly affiliated with a commodification and market logic. As illustrated in the case studies, however, several logics frequently operate simultaneously.

Clearly, gifting is most frequently positioned as separate from the logic of economics and the market logic. In the foreword to Mauss's oft-quoted text *The Gift*, Douglas (1990) forcefully argues that there is no such thing as a free gift: "Even the idea of a pure gift is a contradiction. By ignoring the universal custom of compulsory gifts we

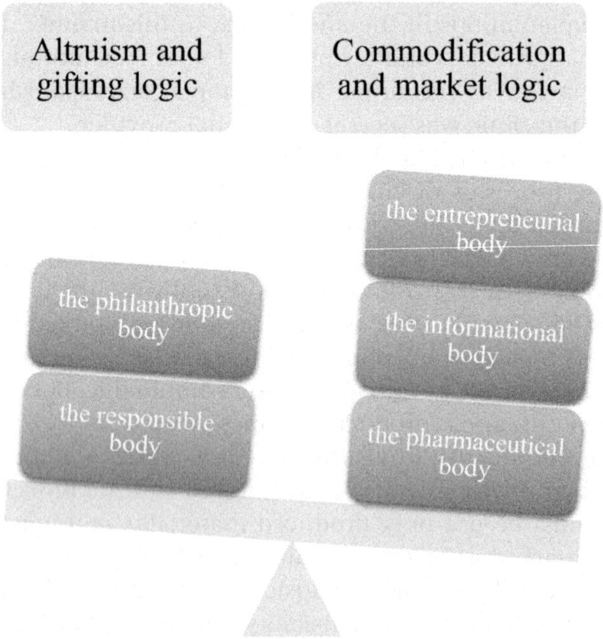

FIGURE 5.1. The altruism/commodification logics revealing the ways that imagined reproductive bodies are produced within each logic yet also how they frequently intersect them.

make our own record incomprehensible to ourselves: right across the globe and as far back as we can go in the history of human civilization, the major transfer of goods has been by cycles of obligatory returns of gifts" (Douglas 1990: x). As also noted by Mauss ([1950] 1990), gifts are given to expand solidarity and the network of social relations. Strathern similarly notes that gifting establishes a relationship between the exchanging subjects (Strathern 1988: 143). However, this is in sharp contrast to the ways that the gift model is structured and managed within the realm of organ procurement and reproduction. In reference to organ procurement, Jackson notes, "Giving of the gift is not grounded in any immediate social relationship between recipients and donor. As such the gift is asocial, and resembles an alienated object, a commodity" (Jackson 2002: 333). Similarly, in his work on egg donation in Spain, Bestard (2004) argues that the very idea of gifting, as it is carried out in the specific context of the Spanish oocyte economy, suppresses the giver in order to grant the receiver the right of kinship:

> In this process the giver is suppressed as a person creating relations; only her eggs are valuable. The receiver on the other hand has the right of kinship because she asked for the services of the reproductive clinic. She has a project of motherhood and will share the biogenetic substance of kinship with her offspring even if biogenetics does not literally mean genetics. The enduring and diffuse solidarity of kinship can be symbolized not only by biological substance, but also by relational actions as desire, gestation and care. (Bestard 2004: 256)

In what follows, I turn to a discussion of the notion of gift markets, delineating feminist interventions in the ways that reproductive donations enter into and exit out of the commodity state, necessitating a discussion of what the market logic does to our understanding of reproductive gifting. I agree with Klaus Hoeyer (2013) that new analytical approaches to the ways that tissues and cells are made to appear exchangeable are sorely needed. As echoed in Hoeyer's (2013) work, the idea of the market is commonly understood as consisting of subjects who have ownership of commodities or objects. This understanding of the market, however, does not adequately capture the empirical complexities or the ways in which global reproductive fluids flow. Rather, Hoeyer (2013) suggests a radical change in vocabulary, which altogether avoids the notion of the "gift" and the "market" and instead employs the vocabulary of "exchange," "ubject," and "entitlement." Whereas the concept of "exchange" is clearly less morally loaded (compared to the word "market"), the term "ubject" is deliberatively, Hoeyer (2013) admits, strange, yet it seeks to disrupt the subject-object divide (persons vs. things). Meanwhile, the term "entitlement" sidesteps "ownership" as a conceptual category (Hoeyer 2013: 4–6). Although Hoeyer (2013) is successful in formulating a new vocabulary for understanding how reproductive fluids enter in and out of exchange situations, for now, I hold on to the notion of "gift markets" to explicitly situate the case studies in relationship to previous feminist scholarship.

Gifts and Markets

Feminist scholars have provided us with sharp analytical insights and historicized reproductive gift markets (Almeling 2009; Dickenson 2009; Sharp 2000; Scheper-Hughes 2015; Strathern 1988). In fact, Strathern highlights the productive tension between the gift and the commodity when she notes that the "prevalence of gift exchange as opposed to one dominated by commodity exchange opens up conceptual possibilities for the language that conceives of a contrast between them" (Strathern 1988: 19). This perspective coincides with Hoeyer's call for a challenge of market thinking, when he notes that empirical analyses reveal when and how things become commodities: "We need to *denaturalize* market thinking as a transparent representation of exchange, while simultaneously taking into account how notions of markets are embedded in very *concrete* experiences and material exchange practices and have performative effects for them" (Hoeyer 2013: 35). In this subsection I follow these theoretical perspectives and depart from the view that reproductive fluids are exclusively either gifts or commodities, at first situating reproduction within the context of feminist accounts and economics and then returning to Strathern's (1988) desire to unfold the gift and commodity tension by asking, what kinds of things are these reproductive donations, and what does the positioning of them as gifts or commodities *do* in terms of what social forms they take?

In feminist accounts, the commodification of women's reproductive abilities and also their parts is situated within the context of late-modern forms of capitalism (DasGupta and Das Dasgupta 2010; Dickenson 2009; Scheper-Hughes 2015). Reproduction is understood as involving gendered understandings of female/male reproductive bodies, as well as being deeply embedded within a class-based and race-based economy, in which younger, less financially secure women become "natural" egg providers while working-class women, sometimes of color, become surrogates. Almeling (2009) illustrates this swiftly in her analyses of the ways in which the contemporary U.S. gamete market is gendered. Whereas egg donation, in spite of high compensation rates, is constructed as an act of altruism, sperm donation is viewed as akin to a job, even in the face of lower and more fixed compensation rates. Consequently, Almeling concludes, "In this market, it is not just reproductive material, but visions of middle-class American femininity and masculinity, and more to the point, of motherhood and fatherhood, that are marketed and purchased" (Almeling 2009: 57).

But what does the IVF (gift) market look like, estimated to exceed US$21 billion globally by 2020 ("Global Fertility Services Market" 2016)? As demonstrated throughout this book, reproductive donations entangle not only with the market in fertility treatments (eggs) but also with the market in beauty, weight loss, and health (placentas and urine), as well as the pharmaceutical market (placentas and urine). In the case of IVF treatments, the market consists of suppliers (e.g., gamete providers, companies specializing in various treatment services, cryopreservation technologies, cryopreservation media), clinics and also customers (frequently positioned as intended parents, clients, or patients), prices (linking supply and demand), and supply routes (including transportation routes). Similarly, the cosmetic and pharmaceutical markets employing placentas or urine as raw resources consist of providers (animals or human providers), pickup services (transportation), processing plants, and consumers (most frequently, women purchasing anti-aging lotions or fertility hormones). Clearly, this is a specialty market, but in many ways it is a very significant market nonetheless. Spar echoes this when she notes, "Harsh as it may seem, we need to view reproductive medicine as an industry, with all of the commercial prospects and potential foibles that other industries display. We also need to look closely at the prices that prevail in this industry and the relationships between various market segments" (Spar 2006: xv).

What does the market logic *do* then to our understanding of reproduction? De-emphasizing gifting and instead understanding IVF and reproductive fluids within the logics of the market and economics makes certain reproductive routes possible and visible. For example, urine is provided to the pharmaceutical industry at no or little cost, and women undergoing IVF, whether as egg providers or recipients, rarely choose their drug of choice but instead buy the drug that the doctor prescribes. Meanwhile, recipients actively choose their clinic of choice, if they can afford it, as does the egg provider. Animal or human placentas enter the beauty and health industries at little cost, yet these are transformed into profitable commodities.

Addressing the processes of commodification, Appadurai notes that commodities are "things in a certain situation," thus specifying the importance of the commodity situation as "*the social life of any 'thing' being defined as the situation in which its exchangeability (past, present, future) for some other thing is its socially relevant feature*" (Appadurai 1986: 13; italics author). Reproductive fluids entangle, in this manner, with the commodity context. In chapter 3, the Danish travelers redefine their entrance into the Spanish clinic of choice as entering a "money machine," while they remain skeptical of the Danish doctor at the private clinic, who has a pronounced tan, signifying not only time but also money to travel. While most of them refuse to view their treatment as "buying the hopes for a child," they capture the services offered by the clinics as deeply embedded in a commodity context. As the empirical examples throughout chapters 2–4 illustrate, "commodification lies at the complex intersection of temporal, cultural and social factors" (Appadurai 1986: 15).

The commodity context, and most notably the effects of it, is heavily criticized in feminist accounts. To transnational feminists, reproductive technologies are stratified markets—built upon existing power hierarchies between women in the western and northern parts of the world and women in the developing countries. As noted by Gupta, transnational feminist analyses must recognize "the fact that one's privileges in the world system are always linked to another woman's oppression or exploitation" (Gupta 2006: 34). This scholarship displays an acute awareness as to how the commodity context plays out differently, including its historical entanglement with stratifications based on gendered and racialized geopolitics. What may have the appearance of an "egalitarian swap" (DasGupta and Das Dasgupta 2010: 141), in which infertile Westerners gain a child and motherhood in exchange for economic resources, is instead a reiteration of a particular, gendered political landscape, in which particular women (frequently third-world, less economically privileged women) become gift-giving providers while other women are "naturally" situated as gift recipients (frequently first-world, more economically privileged women).

In this manner, feminist scholars direct our attention to the ways in which the market logic in reproduction reiterates gendered and raced understandings of desirable bodies, as well as able-bodied, flawless, "own" children (Colen 1995; Ginsburg and Rapp 1995). Addressing the specific issue of race and desire, Nahman (2008, 2006) illustrates how whiteness becomes a trait selected by intending Israeli parents while the Romanian donor's economic marginality makes the exchanges possible in the first place. The commodification of sperm serves as another case in point. As argued by Daniels and Golden (2004), sperm is not only tested and screened to ensure a healthy bioproduct, but it is also, most notably, marketed according to particular social desires (e.g., tall, young, intelligent, sociable, and attractive sperm), reinforcing the idea that physical and even social traits are genetic and heritable. Daniels and Golden summarize the commodification of sperm as follows: "What consumers want to buy is more than a means of remedying nature's unfairness, they want to buy what they perceive to be the best that nature and science can, together, provide" (Daniels and Golden 2004: 12). In a similar vein, Kroløkke (2009) analyzes the marketing and branding of Danish sperm as "Viking" sperm and shows how it is reconfigured into a healthy, outgoing, robust, athletic, and attractive commodity, in which race and location are conflated to produce the notion of Scandinavian men as innately blond, healthy, athletic, and white.

In the market logic, race and nationality entangle with reproductive fluids in several ways. Not only are gametes neatly "packaged" into white, Asian, black, and mix-raced sperm and eggs (Russell 2015), race also infiltrates the gift market in reproduction and medically assisted reproduction in other ways. In critiquing the notion of "race science" and instead suggesting "race idea" as a term, Russell (2015) shows how race is present in clinical practices (for example, in the overview of the international clients in the Spanish fertility clinic), gets intertwined with social imaginaries on who is fit to parent, reappears when (and in what geographical locations) (in)fertility is considered a problem, and works by making racial sameness in cases of IVF appear as desirable—even normal. The race idea functions, Russell (2015) argues, by re-naturalizing conventional understandings of racial separation and difference. Similarly, in the clinical practices in Spain as well as in Denmark, clinicians go to great lengths to ensure that no racial "mix-up" takes place, and when they do take place, racial discrimination—rather than the whiteness of the ART system itself—gets the blame. This is, for example, present in a well-publicized Danish case in which a white Danish couple going through IVF mistakenly received the wrong embryo (that of an Iranian woman and a sperm provider). And it is also present in the Spanish clinic when egg providers from South America have to detail the race of grandparents as well as great-grandparents (unlike the single generation that the Russian egg providers have to describe). In this manner, the race idea underlies the particular reproductive paths that the South American provider (unlike the Russian provider) has to undergo.

As evident in the case studies, the gift-market logic is raced and classed in other ways as well. Returning to Cohen's (2005) theoretical framework of bioavailability and supplementarity, for example, we see how women's bodies and reproductive fluids entangle with the market in reproduction. For example, oocytes are made to appear bioavailable, yet the ease with which oocytes are made available, and at times move, is frequently the result of intersectional power dynamics, including East-West hierarchies in which (some) women's bodies are naturalized as more available than some (other) women's bodies. In the case of oocytes and the discussion in chapter 3, this pertained especially to younger, white, less economically privileged, migrant women. Vora (2015) echoes this in her analysis of transnational surrogacy in which Indian women are made to appear available to women and men from the Global North. Bioavailability entangles, in this manner, with race and nationality, while the concept of supplementarity, defined as "the ability of an individual or population to be able to mobilize such a flow of organic form toward itself" (Cohen 2005: 32), critically interrogates the directionality of this reproductive flow. In chapter 3, Northern European women rationalized and naturalized their desire for pregnancy and motherhood in their travel to Spain, while also in this chapter, traveling egg providers from the Global North rationalized their decision to provide other women with their genetic material through an upward desire to travel and give the gift of fertility.

While the categories of race, nationality, gender, and class clearly entangle in the gift-market framework, they are, as evident in the case studies, frequently made to appear invisible. Instead, commodification is transformed into a logic of reusability and extensibility of the female (reproductive) body's economic potential. In the case of oocytes (chapter 3), eggs are seen as "going to waste" (when unused or aging). Meanwhile, in the case of urine, peeing into a bottle and handing it over to the fertility industry gets reframed as giving another woman "the gift of love" (chapter 2). Once urine enters the pharmaceutical industry, however, it quickly departs the glorified frame of a "love commodity" and turns into a hormone treatment or a pregnancy test, sold and marketed to medical professionals contributing to the transnational pharmaceutical industry as well as women's reliance of the pregnancy test as a self-testing technology. Similarly, the whitewashing of Danish porcine placentas that unfolds in the Japanese pharmaceutical industry secures a particular understanding of this raw material as promoting hygiene and health, yet now frozen, processed, and flown to Japan. While the reproductive donations circulate in very different ways, they jointly contribute to the financial viability of the international fertility and pharmaceutical industry.

Within the gift-market logic, the reproductive body is frequently viewed as a fragmented and fragmentary body. Moreover, when commodification unfolds, it has the effect of making certain decisions and routes legitimate, as also noted by Cohen (2005), and the desire for particular types of characteristics appears just, even natural. Sharp criticizes this as an act of dehumanization when, in reference to the effects of commodification, she says, "Commodification insists upon objectification in some form, transforming persons and their bodies from a human category into objects of economic desire" (Sharp 2000: 293). The British 2002 example serves as a case in point. Here, two university students were paid to travel to California to provide their eggs to two different women, at the prices of £3,800 and £5,000 respectively. While the amount is not outstanding compared to elite egg provider practices in the United States, the comment made by Karen Synesiou, the director of the Center for Surrogate Parenting, Inc. testifies to the way that certain bodies are made to appear available for reproductive consumption: "If you're not attractive, you're not going to get anywhere in egg donation. Nobody wants an ugly child if they can help it," Synesiou reportedly said.[1] In this context, commodification is seen to depersonalize and dehumanize the body according to Sharp (2000). Hoeyer (2013) echoes this logic as well when he notes, "If an object of human dignity becomes tradable, it is transformed into something of lower moral standing" (Hoeyer 2013: 18).

When viewed as commodities, however, reproductive fluids are "objects with self-contained value, capable of being owned and circulated as property, without reference to the social sources of production" (Strathern 1988: 152). While placentas and urine clearly have the capacity to turn into vital ingredients in new products and commodities that bear little trace, if any, of the respective providers or their original state, women's oocytes, in the empirical material discussed in chapter 3, bear traces to the women (or the country) they came from. While pluripotent, they are only capable of being used once. Whereas the commodity label has the effect of separating the provider (e.g., the urine and placenta provider) from the product (the pills or the lotion), the choice to position these interactions as anonymous gift exchanges does little to extend social relationships between particular women and particular recipients. Rather, in the words of Fox and Swazey (1992), reproductive fluids undergo a process of de-gifting that enables new entanglements to occur. The combination of gifting with anonymity and a market that systematically categorizes reproductive donations in light of various qualities (dark haired, athletic, student representative, a great mother) makes reproductive fluids, at least in the case of eggs, seem to "naturally" belong to the recipient woman, raising issues related to the property rights, if any, that these fluids hold.

Objects without Owners

Following the birth of her baby, Jordan Thiering, a pregnant resident of Mississippi, went through the state courts in the spring of 2016 in order to be granted the rights to her own placenta. Planning to take the placenta home, she checked the hospital rules and regulations, only to learn, much to her surprise, that she needed a court order to get the right to dispose of the placenta: "I'm thinking, 'What? For my own body part? Why do I need a court order?'" (Staff 2016). According to the Mississippi Department of Health, Thiering was a third party to her placenta. Fortunately, at thirty-three weeks pregnant, she received the court order. Most people would be surprised to learn that the placenta was not Thiering's to take home. It was not her property. Bodies and body parts are not properties, yet developments in medical technologies call for new proprietary rights in the body (Dickenson 2002; Strathern 1999; Knaplund 2004). This is seen in other cases as well, such as the 2015 California case in which a divorced couple took their disagreement over their stored and frozen embryos—which had been frozen during their marriage as a result of the woman's earlier battle with breast cancer and subsequent treatment—to court (Hill 2015). The judge ruled in favor of the ex-husband, denying the woman the ability to use the embryos in medically assisted reproduction.

What these cases have in common is a set of missing property rights (Dickenson 2002; Strathern 1999; Knaplund 2004; Spar 2006). In the Thiering case, if the placenta was not hers as afterbirth matter, then whose was it? Upon expulsion, did it then belong to no one? Was it the newborn baby's property, or perhaps the hospital's? In the example of the divorced couple, the Findley v. Lee case, the embryos consisted of reproductive material from both partners, intended for use by the couple in medically assisted reproduction. In this case, the judge employed a contractual model to prioritize the ex-husband's reproductive autonomy at the expense of the ex-wife's reproductive abilities, stating his unwillingness to enact court-ordered fatherhood. In this subsection I turn to feminist legal and sociological scholarship to discuss what I term reproductive objects without owners. I then proceed by analyzing how the informed consent form functions as a very specific disentanglement tool, managing and resolving the question of property in the body in order to procure, store, process, and market reproductive fluids.

Clearly, the notion of property in the body is contentious, at a minimum. To legal scholars, property is usually granted, Skene (2012) argues, through the lawful exercise of work and skill. A property interest can, however, arise in something that was not previously property (Skene 2012). Because we have not labored to create our own bodies, we do not have any property rights in our bodies and thus, the notion of property in the body is an oxymoron at best, Dickenson (2007) argues. This is especially the case with bodily extracts. They are positioned as res nullius—belonging to no one—yet importantly, when reappropriated, they are able to become the property of someone else. Now, the fact that property in the body is disputed and the trading in other people's bodies is illegal does not mean that individuals do not make decisions on their own bodies. As argued by Strathern (1988), ownership is linked to the idea that individuals are the authors of their own thoughts and actions. Consequently, we govern our own actions, but the legal right is not extended to the individual, for example, to sell a kidney, rent out a womb for surrogacy, or sell a placenta. Phillips echoes this and says: "The body *is* yours, but that does not make it property, and does not give you the automatic right to determine to rent out or sell" (Phillips 2013: 3). This particular understanding of property in the body is echoed in Danish bioethical accounts, in which bodily properties entangle with commodification to produce what becomes constructed as a loss of human dignity, resulting in human objects that are turned into tradable objects.[2]

What does this notion of property in the body do to the circulation of reproductive fluids? Clearly, human bodies and human body parts cannot be traded or sold yet, even though I have repeatedly demonstrated in this book that they continually are. Gametes and organs are examples of parts that circulate against the payment of a fee, typically reframed as compensation. Moreover, the pharmaceutical industry and the burgeoning IVF industry strongly testify to the fact that there is a market in (the making of) children. The use of reproductive bodies and their parts extends far beyond the reproductive realm. This is especially clear when considering reproduction in terms of the larger realm of working, laboring, productive bodies. Productive bodies have already been used and exploited in the name of nationalism and the development of Gross National Product (GNP). For instance, take the case of factory workers around the globe who use their bodies to manufacture products that are sold elsewhere. Similarly, skilled as well as unskilled laborers use their bodies in the military, in mines, and in the construction industry to produce safety and wealth for others. What these cases have in common is the fact that workers use their bodies within the realm of production. So why does putting the "re-" into the productive body become so controversial? To the cultural analyst, property language does something when applied within the gendered sphere of reproduction. It not only positions the reproductive body and children as metaphorical and literal commodities but it also genders reproduction and consequently scrutinizes and disciplines the reproductive actors within it. In the Danish case, sperm-providing is celebrated as a Danish export commodity, while oocyte-providing, when entangled with the world of compensation, frequently gets seen as worrisome and is then considered as a potential form of trafficking and reproductive exploitation.

Reproductive property rights frequently coincide with rhetoric on "choice" and thus ideas on reproductive autonomy (Petchesky 1995). As echoed by Hayden and Hallstein, choice suggests rational deliberation (Hayden and Hallstein 2010: xvii). However, choice is also highly individualized and stratified. Phillips notes this about reproductive choice and property, within the specific context of commercial surrogacy, when she says that the rhetoric of choice only "solves the problem of infertility if we limit our definition of the infertile to those who can afford to pay" (Phillips 2013: 154). Choice is here a choice in disguise, and consequently, at least to some, no choice at all. Strathern echoes this when she notes that choosing becomes a sign of active citizenship, in which individuals have the choice to choose responsibly, or, as presented by her, "The exercise of choice that defines the active citizen is market choice, not just because of the kinds of rules of the game associated with free bargaining or an equation between enterprising selves and business enterprise, but because the market also deals in things which have been market*ed*" (Strathern 1992: 38). Egg freezing is a testament to this. While freezing one's eggs gets promoted as a form of gender equality—enhancing women's reproductive choices—egg freezing can also be viewed as a form of compulsory heterosexuality and self-responsibility, ensuring one's reproductive abilities and consequently optimizing one's attractiveness in a culture that promotes reproduction and the making of own children. As noted by Strathern, in the enterprise culture, one's choices must always be self-enhancing (Strathern 1992: 37). And similarly, Lemke notes that neoliberal governmentality calls for "prudent subjects whose moral quality is based on the fact that they rationally assess the costs and benefits of a certain act as opposed to other alternative acts" (Lemke 2001: 201).

As a technology, the informed consent form manages reproductive property. According to Callon (1998) and Dickenson (2007), the form settles the exchange of reproductive entitlements. It can aptly be viewed as a very specific type of disentanglement that effectively separates reproductive tissue and fluids from the bodies they came from. Dickenson views the informed consent form akin to this, yet also repositions it into a cover-up for one-way altruism: "Whereas the original purpose of gift, in the anthropological literature, is to establish ongoing relationships of indebtedness and gratitude that binds societies together, the intent of some current guidelines seems to be the exact opposite: to cut off any further claims by the donor and any continuing obligations for the clinician, researcher or biotechnology corporation in receipt of the gift" (Dickenson 2007: 18). Similarly, Cooper and Waldby position the informed consent form as enabling specific forms of unequal exchanges, while they note that the reproductive contract specifies property rights and reproductive entitlements as always being already within the confines of the recipient couple (Cooper and Waldby 2014). To this extent, the informed consent form, along with the reproductive contract (egg provider contract, for example), serve very particular purposes and forms of reproductive intent.

In combination, the informed consent form and the contract make particular reproductive routes accessible, even imaginable. Both forms work to ensure the "rightful" exchange in reproductive entitlements, yet they are not without their own sets of problems. Consider, for example, the case in the United Kingdom in which new mothers initially gave their consent for their placentas to be used for research, only to learn later that they were used in research benefitting the cosmetic industry (mentioned in chapter 4). One placenta provider stressed her confusion when she reportedly said, "I was under the impression that my placenta would only be used for vital medical research—not that it may help make some skin cream or shampoo." Another reckons, "They said my placenta would be used to help research to cure cancer. They didn't mention anything else. I was elated having just given birth and just signed it" (Sawer 2008).[3] While the consent form ensures that the provider waives her future rights and potential entitlements of ownership, the actual reproductive paths undertaken may conflict with the stipulated paths, as well as those imagined by the providers. Moreover, the value of the reproductive donation emerges out of various entangled and embodied social relationships. The egg can be disentangled, creating a transmutation in value from having investment value (as frozen oocytes) to having scientific potential (in the stem cell industry as future value), to having market value (as donated oocytes), or as having no value (as waste and accordingly discarded by its owner, or more likely the clinic). Thus, through the consent form as a property instrument, reproductive donations entangle with personal, scientific, and market values.

The empirical material and the analyses presented in chapters 2–4 suggest a need to rethink the meanings of reproductive property and ownership. As noted by Petchesky, the notion of private property refers to things that are owned, as well as the right to keep others out: "This relational basis of property adheres despite our culturally induced propensity to translate rights of access into objects of exchange" (Petchesky 1995: 389). Moreover, property is a discursive construction emphasizing that women have "authority over" their reproductive parts and fluids (Petchesky 1995: 403). Chapter 4 revealed several examples of women using their placentas as forms of gender empowerment, while elective freezers in chapter 3 exerted agency in freezing their reproductive material for potential future use, including strengthening their position in a competitive urban dating market. As noted in these analyses, property rights are not without their sets of problems. Whereas property rights over the placenta enable women to consume or dispose of the placenta as they see fit, they are also a very particular gendered type of enactment. Similarly, the purported agency associated with freezing one's reproductive potential not only positions women as responsible for reproduction (in contrast to more structural levels of responsibility) but also creates new positions of future IVF consumers, as frozen eggs can only be used through the mechanisms of IVF.

Having discussed legal and sociological perspectives on the enactment of property rights, including the informed consent form, I now turn to the ways that these reproductive flows are contingent upon what I refer to as waste management labor.

Waste Management Labor: Philanthropy Meets Entrepreneurship

Because reproductive fluids do not appear out of nowhere, I return in this section to the imagined reproductive bodies (chapters 2–4), and I discuss the work that goes into making and processing global fluids. Throughout I apply the term "regenerative labor" (Cooper and Waldby 2014) to explain the work that goes into the making or providing of these fluids. The choice to use "regenerative" as a term is done, akin to Cooper and Waldby (2014), to suggest that women's reproductive work has transformative value: reproductive donations move from the home, the fertility clinic, or the birthing clinic and into the fertility clinic, processing plants, the hormone industry, or the cosmetic industry, for example. Therefore, as a term, "regenerative" suggests that the transformative value inherent in these reproductive fluids extends beyond the immediate reproductive potential. Moreover, the term "labor" is used, as Cooper and Waldby (2014) reckon, to conjure up different meanings: women "go into" labor when they give birth, and workers labor to produce (Cooper and Waldby 2014: 33).

Consequently, in upholding the concept of "regenerative labor," two meanings are suggested: not only do women labor to produce eggs (through hormone injections), urine (through bottling and pouring the fluid), and placentas (through pushing), but women also enact the positions of laborers in these commodity situations. So the decision to view the work that goes into reproductive fluids as a type of regenerative labor can aptly be seen in relationship to that of the self-made, entrepreneurial woman. To Rose, individuals become "entrepreneurs of themselves, shaping their own lives through the choices they make among the forms of life available to them" (Rose 1999: 230). Within the realm of transnational reproduction, Kroløkke (2012, 2015) notes that terms such as "eggpreneur" and "repropreneur" jointly speak to egg-donor mobility, as well as the ways that the decision to become a reproductive laborer, when mixed with neoliberal ideologies, draws on entrepreneurial qualities and discourses. A central argument in these contributions has been that repro-entrepreneurship is positioned jointly within a moral economy of gifting and neoliberal ideology. Traveling to provide other women with eggs, or the decision to become a surrogate, must be understood within an affective economy of upward mobility. In both cases, neoliberal ideology functions as a model of action based on economic entrepreneurship, in which reproductive citizens are transformed into active "repropreneurs"—the mobile reproductive clients/consumers/assistants/workers of a global economy in reproductive services (Kroløkke and Pant 2012). Pollock echoes this complexity in her ethnographic study on egg providers when she notes that they "are free enough to be complicit in a process that exploits them as they seek their own rewards" (Pollock 2003: 247).

In this manner, women's regenerative labor can be viewed as both disentangled and an affective type of labor. Callon (1998) argues that disentanglements are necessary for reproductive donations to circulate in the first place. Not in reference to reproduction, but in more general terms, Callon says, "If the thing remains entangled, the one who receives is never able to quit and cannot escape from the web of relations" (Callon 1998: 19). In fact, Dickenson offers us a feminist critique when, in relation to women's labor within egg providing, she argues that "women's labor in producing oocytes for private IVF clinics and the stem cell technologies has brought the most intimate, 'archaic' biological functions into the marketplace" (Dickenson 2007: 53). Feminist scholars acknowledge the ways that, in their enactments of regenerative work, women are both disentangled from the realm of work and also, in concrete clinical practices, re-entangled into a gift economy.

A central argument of this book has been that the work that goes into urine, egg, and placenta providing is productive as well as reproductive. Dickenson points to the effects of this when she comments that "the effect of the new biotechnologies is to take the propertylessness in the labor of reproduction back to stages before the birth of children" (Dickenson 2007: 54). Thus, while women's work within the home as well as in the sphere of reproduction has frequently been excluded from the realm of value (as non-labor), feminist scholars have successfully demonstrated how women's labor (pregnancy, childbirth, ova production, homemaking, etc.) is economic in nature. Separated from the notion of paid public labor, the reproductive work undertaken by urine, egg, and placenta providers re-entangles with notions of mothering, positioned by Dickenson as forms of "home production" (Dickenson 2007: 56). Providing others with urine, eggs, and placentas in this manner is an act of (re)productive work. For instance, the work that goes into placenta preparation and consumption can be considered as a very specific type of maternal work done to ensure the surplus energy needed to fulfill other maternal obligations. Similarly, administering the hormone shots involved in the process of egg providing is a very specific type of routinized work that requires disciplined, responsible female bodies.

Linking commodification, labor and capitalism within the context of (re)production, I will briefly turn to the Marxian concept of alienation. Once again, the work undertaken by Dickenson is useful. According to her, "If reproductive labor in the home can be viewed as alienated, then certainly alienation can apply to reproductive labor undertaken outside the home, and to a situation where there need be no inverted commas around 'product.' Although children are neither property nor truly a product, stem cells are both" (Dickenson 2007: 76). Whereas Dickenson's focus is on the use of ova in the stem cell industry, the same argument can be made about the labor that goes into urine and placenta providing and, importantly, the work that goes into the production of hormone replacement therapies or anti-aging, whitening lotions. Moreover, the fact that providers of urine, eggs and placentas are frequently nameless and always women contributes to this potential lack of acknowledgment. Ova, urine, and placentas unfold in gendered milieus that frequently benefit recipients, companies, clinics, as well as academic and industrial venues. As echoed in feminist scholarship, the fact that reproductive tissue and fluids can be developed, extracted, retrieved, stored, thawed, and eventually created into new products that are put up for sale does not mean that women actually benefit from these transactions (Dickenson 2002).

Regenerative labor is viewed as not merely physical in nature—it is highly affective as well. Similar to Ahmed (2004), I pose that emotions mediate the relationship between the provider and the recipient in a particular way, securing the recipient's rights to kinship while also re-aligning reproductive donations to particular and frequently heteronormative ideologies. From a sociological point of view, Hochschild (1979) critically interrogates the commodification of feelings as gendered and classed. As she notes in her critique of the service industry dominated by young female workers, "There are jobs, like that of secretary or airline stewardess, with relatively low financial rewards and little authority, which nonetheless require a high degree of emotion and display management. Such jobs are often filled by women, many of whom come from the middle class" (Hochschild 1979: 570). In the case of egg providing, women are scrutinized for their ability to perform a very particular type of femininity. Pollock demonstrates this in her work, when egg providers enact acceptable forms of femininity: "In order to be an egg donor, a woman must perform a coherent representation of a normal self" (Pollock 2003: 258). The "good" egg provider enacts altruism and ideal notions of femininity in giving other women a chance at motherhood. Similarly, the "good" urine provider enacts the philanthropic reproductive body, which happily participates to ensure another woman's (naturalized) desire for motherhood, despite the smell, the outing of one's pregnancy to a curious neighbor, and the inconvenience. In these performances, urine and egg providers signal a definition of self as "caring" and "reliable," consistent with Hochchild's (1979) emotion rules and illustrative of the ways that emotions also become properties. This is in sharp contrast to the entrepreneurial provider body departing from gendered expectations of women being closely attached to their reproductive fluids and thus, in some sense, challenges whitewashed gendered norms of women's reproductive agency as exclusively tied to a logic of gifting.

The waste management labor that goes into these reproductive donations must be seen as normative, as well as enacted through the employment of highly standardized, routinized practices. Hogle argues that standardized practices ensure the management of social relationships, including the reconstruction of how reproductive fluids should be used (Hogle 1995: 483). In the Danish public birthing clinics, routinized practices ensure that placentas move from the birthing woman to the incinerator. Not surprisingly, few Danish women (if any) within the public clinic ever ask to take the placenta home. While the midwives display the placenta for the new parents to see, enabling them to photograph it if they so wish, they ensure that their own reproductive practices involved in weighing and scrutinizing the placenta, as well as bagging it in the yellow bag, largely go unnoticed. Hogle (1995) says that these routinized practices discipline how reproductive donations can move, in the process disentangling and re-entangling reproductive fluids as naturally belonging to someone or somewhere else.

Having briefly presented the reproductive work that goes into reproductive fluids, I will now turn to a discussion of the cultural politics of reproductive fluids.

A Repro-Politics of Reusability and Extensibility

This book has had two agendas: First, it has sought to explore how reproductive fluids transition from waste to value. Reproductive fluids move from individual bodies to storage and processing facilities, laboratories, fertility clinics, birthing clinics, and freezing tanks, while they are simultaneously reimagined in advertisements, films, and social media, turned into products and brands that are consumed by hopeful female (reproductive) bodies. And second, this book has attempted to develop and discuss a feminist cultural politics of reproduction in which the "global" and the "fluid" become analytical incisions and empirically forefront the practices and ways that urine, placentas, and eggs move in the imagination of individual women, in marketing material, in clinical practices, and also in industrial processes. In fact, from a feminist bioethical point of view, Shildrick suggests that "leakiness" may deconstruct categories and demonstrate "the inescapability of the leaks and flows across all such bodies of knowledge and bodies of matter" (Shildrick 1997: 4). In this final section of the conclusion, I highlight this latter agenda by discussing how a cultural politics of reusability and extensibility may aptly frame the various dis- and re-entanglements that reproductive fluids undergo throughout their circulations and cultural imaginaries.

But first, a return to the ways that reproductive fluids can be seen as global is in order. At first glance, reproductive fluids appear as distinctly localized matter and practices. The placenta exits the birthing body as a localized fleshy and bloody reproductive organ. Similarly, urine splashes into a pitcher, later to be transferred into a container residing inside or outside the provider's home. In chapter 1, I referred to the global in two ways: as a form of network and also, more metaphorically, as a fluid (Urry 2000). When understood as a network, the global involves mapping the ways that providers, patients, consumers, clients, factories, and clinics are interlinked. Urine is provided by individual pregnant women to Moeders voor Moeders in the Netherlands, transported to the factory, reassembled into powder or injections, shipped to pharmacies and doctors around the world, and then prescribed to and purchased by patients on the global stage. Similarly, through their affiliations with a Danish private clinic, Danish women in need of eggs may travel to clinics in Spain, Greece, the Ukraine, or Russia. Egg providers travel transnationally to a network of clinics located in the United States, Cyprus, South Africa, and Barbados, for example, and large fertility clinics not only create routinized fertility care in Spain but are also expanding through franchising to Argentina, Brazil, Chile, Portugal, Panama, and Mexico. Meanwhile, Danish women may choose to photograph the placenta, bring it home, cook it, and later eat it. On a much more global scale, the placentas of Danish pigs are refrigerated, picked up, and sent to Japan as a necessary ingredient in anti-aging lotions. These networks are decidedly global, as they feature entanglements of reproductive bodies, factories, farmers, and clinics that crisscross national, legal, and ethical boundaries.

When the global is understood in the second meaning of the term—as a fluid—it is understood as having "heterogeneous, uneven and unpredictable mobilities," as argued by Urry (2000: 38). Leaky bodies threaten to disturb the patriarchal order: "Just as the excessive and leaky female body threatens self-certainty, so too the leaky logos undermine ontological and epistemological closure" (Shildrick 1997: 104). As noted by Urry (2000), fluids may move in particular directions and at certain speeds, but they do not always keep within the spaces relegated to them and may seep through the walls intended to contain them: they "do not always keep within the walls—they may move outside or escape like white blood corpuscles though the 'wall' of the scape into tinier and tinier caterpillars" (Urry 2000: 39). Here the analytical and empirical interests rest with the ways that the global entangles, as well as disentangles and re-entangles, with localized practices and with particular bodies. Scholars may turn to what Urry calls "globalized empty meeting grounds" (Urry 2000: 39). In the case of reproduction, this includes the waiting room in the global fertility clinic, where women and men, who have flown from around the world, are waiting with the globalized hope for a baby in their own future reproductive mobility (Kroløkke 2016); this also includes how the logics acquired in the IVF laboratories of human and animal embryo transfers come to take up global form (Knecht et al. 2012) and constitute globalized understandings of reproductive routines applicable to clinics across the globe (Franklin 2005).

As a metaphor, the global must be understood critically as well. As noted by Franklin et al., in their formulation of a feminist cultural analytical perspective, the global is a "fantasy, a set of practices," a "set of effects" and also "an aspiration rather than an achievement" (Franklin et al. 2000: 5). Based on Ingold's (1993) discussion of the iconic power of the globe and its place in the cultural imaginary of the global, Urry, moreover, notes how this perspective on the globe (and the global) promotes a "global ontology of detachment over the local ontology of engagement—it is to celebrate technology, intervention, expert management and the relative disempowerment of the local people" (Urry 2000: 46). Urry (2000) argues that not only is the dichotomy between the global and the local frequently reiterated, but this understanding of the global also fails to critique the metaphor of the global as being removed from localized practices, yet frequently it also ends up repositioning local practices as more "real." In this book I have understood the global as well as the local as *enactments* with performative effects and as cultural imaginaries, or as noted by Franklin et al., the global can also be understood as a "discursive condition," positioned as an effect as much as a condition (Franklin et al. 2000: 4, 5).

Throughout the book, reproductive donations have been viewed as global *fluids*. In using "fluid" as a term, I have relied on Mol and Law's (1994) notion that "fluids" escape boundaries, have no particular pathways, and have to be understood not exclusively as networks but rather as sets of relations that come together to form a flow: "The study of fluids, then, will be a study of the relations, repulsions and attractions which form a flow. Repulsions, which sometimes, to be sure, mean that a fluid encounters its limits" (Mol and Law 1994: 664). At times, reproductive fluids flow to acquire commodity status, understood by Lash and Lury as "goods [that] are commodities to the extent that they exchange, not for other goods, but for money, for units of abstract equivalence on markets" (Lash and Lury 2007: 6). In the case of reproductive fluids covered in this book, compensation is exchanged between providers and clinics (for eggs and porcine placentas), while small gifts characterize the ways that urine flows. Meanwhile, raw material is extracted, exchanged, and made into ingredients or sellable products (in the case of urine and placentas) and sold later at a price (but without compensation to the placenta provider). In spite of these obvious exchanges, reproductive fluids depart from the commodity state in several significant ways. Consequently, more is at stake in understanding the ways that reproductive waste moves and gets fluidic in its exchanges, both locally and also globally.

Through the processes of globalization and the strategies of disentanglement and re-entanglement, global fluids move beyond the commodity state and acquire brand-like and asset-like characteristics. As noted by Lash and Lury (2007) in their analyses of global culture industries, brands acquire value in their distinctiveness to other brands. Consider the cases involving the imagined Spanish eggs mentioned in chapter 3. Here, the provider origin came to constitute quality and superior reproductive material, enticing Danish women to follow reproductive paths to Spain. Similarly, in chapter 2, I illustrated how the afterbirth of Danish pigs is refrigerated, processed, and then shipped to Japan to enter various cosmetic and health-related products. Danish pigs have come to be understood as quality, even healthier than humans living in densely populated

Japanese cities. This branding of Danish reproductive matter is not new. Danish sperm—whether human or animal—is narrated as potent, attractive, healthy, productive, and even robust reproductive matter (Kroløkke 2009). For example, this is evident in the marketing material of one of the world's largest breeding companies owned by farmers and offices in Denmark, Sweden, and Finland. Viking Genetics poses that "the breeding goal for VikingJersey is healthy cows with good fertility, functional conformation and high production."[4] In this manner, reproduction and the geopolitics of health intersect to make reproductive matter brand-like—it becomes "Viking quality." In the meantime, global flows and the ways in which reproductive matter is mediated naturalize particular re-entanglements. As noted in the Danish popular press, in response to business agreements between Thai farmers and Viking Genetics, "The best cow is created through mixing Thai and Danish cows. Whereas the Danish cows are robust, Thai cows are used to the heat" (Nielsen 2014). A somewhat similar picture emerges in the interviews with Danish women who travel to Spain for treatment, in which the provider egg is understood as a "spare part" necessary in the making of "own" children. Consequently, in the "flux and flow of globalization" (Lash and Lury 2007: 9), particular reproductive routes are made to appear possible, drawing on conventional understandings of gender, race, and nationality and thus assisting in moving reproductive donations out of their commodity state to the realm of brands.

Reproductive waste is given new life beyond its value as consumable, marketable, edible, and investable material. In the case of egg freezing, for instance, frozen oocytes entangle with fears of future reproductive failure, as waste-in-the-making yet also as a hopeful reproductive temporality and the making of future babies. In this manner, freezing technologies are depicted as a "natural" technological intervention or assistance. Additionally, reproductive waste gains speculative and asset-like value. This is aptly illustrated in the analyses of eggs and placentas that are both frozen and stored in the fertility clinic, or in the biobank, for potential later use. Theorizing asset-based economic exchanges, Birch and Tyfield (2012) argue for a move from commodity-based processes (e.g., involving production and labor) to more asset-based processes. To Birch, this process is best described as one of assetization in which "value is constituted by the management of value and valuation" (Birch 2017: 470). Value, as defined here by Birch (2017), does not reside in any given thing, but, rather, value accumulates on the basis of the social practices that unfold in particular organizational settings. In chapter 3, the reproductive value inherent in a provider egg was managed by making it valueless or waste-in-the-making, marking its departure from a particular provider body and reassembling it, within the context of the receiver, into valuable genetic matter and a future *own* child. Similarly, the reproductive value of frozen eggs becomes re-temporalized (Franklin 1997), arrested in time and space—promising the provider future reproductive mobility, not only as a mother but also as a marriageable body. Similar to this, and in the case of encapsulation practices mentioned in chapter 4, the placenta escapes the incinerator and is reassembled as hope for good maternity, for an investment in the future health of the genetic family, or for the promise of upward mobility with various beauty transformations involving white, blemish-free skin and silky hair.

As this book draws upon material from vastly different national contexts, it is situated both within transnational gender and reproductive politics and also, at times, within the biopolitics of the welfare state and the rise of neoliberalism. According to Ginsburg and Rapp, a cultural politics of reproduction must recognize this larger geopolitical framework: "In a world in which contests over gender relations, population control, eugenics and opposition to Western imperialism are often seriously interconnected and muddled, the 'politics of reproduction' cannot and should not be extracted from the examination of politics in general" (Ginsburg and Rapp 1991: 331). Similarly, the analyses that have been carried out throughout the chapters in this book have revealed how a cultural politics on reproduction entangles with the state and, in the specific case of the welfare state, the obligation to produce more responsible (tax-paying) citizens (as evidenced in chapter 2 in the attempts to recruit more urine providers). By moving in and out of different reproductive donations, national contexts, and political domains, the three case studies contribute to transnational academic debates on the gendering of the repro-economy, including the development of a cultural politics of reusability and extensibility to which I now turn.

In this last part of the book, I suggest a cultural or repro-politics of reusability and extensibility. In moving the concepts of reusability and extensibility out of the fields of computer and information sciences, where they refer to the ability to use existing assets in the same form as well as the ability to embed possibilities for future growth, I argue that feminist cultural politics must develop concepts that embrace the ways that globalized reproductive fluids entangle with both welfare state and market logics. As Cooper (2008) notes, in the welfare state, the reproductive citizen must dutifully manage her reproductive citizenship in order to reproduce not only the family but the nation. With the rise of neoliberalism, however, reproduction now entangles with the market, fueling the autonomous reproductive citizen as well as speculative biotech markets. In the case chapters, women manage their reproductive flows by optimizing their reusability. For example, while some women are recruited to reuse their oocytes in the context of the fertility industry, other women (who can afford it) naturalize banking their oocytes to ensure their own future genetic reusability. Pregnant women pee in pitchers in the name of Dutch sister solidarity and readily deliver the smelly substance to the MvM organization, while the placenta is gaining new value as an extensible postpartum energizer or an anti-aging ingredient. The logic of reusability and extensibility unfolds not only in clinical practices and within welfare state and capitalist logics more generally, but it is also, as demonstrated throughout this book, taken up by women themselves, frequently entangled with the notion of women *responsibly* and *flexibly* managing their reproductive *autonomy*. Consequently, a cultural politics of reusability and extensibility frame how reproductive fluids depart the category of waste and become valuable, as well as the ways that reproductive autonomy (Denbow 2015) and flexibility (Martin 1994) shape how women's bodies are constructed in a neoliberal and biomedical mode of reproduction (Thompson 2005; Clarke et al. 2010). This includes, but is not limited to, freezing one's oocytes for later use, eating the placenta to gain postpartum energy, and carefully managing one's urine to engage in the nationalized moral citizenship of donating what otherwise may have the appearance of waste.

As cultural tropes, then, reusability and extensibility work across different scales while entangling with cultural expectations of responsible, autonomous, and flexible female reproductive citizens. Whereas the requirement to enact responsible reproductive citizenship has become an earmark of the good female citizenship (Carroll and Kroløkke 2017), autonomy is positioned as a tool for "self-governance" (Denbow 2015: 179), blurring the boundaries between what is considered within the realm of private reproductive decision-making and within the possibilities of intense public scrutiny. As echoed by Martin (1994), the quest to be flexible is everywhere. A cultural politics of usability and extensibility helps frame the ways that the reproductive fluids of urine, eggs, and placentas dis- and re-entangle with women's reproductive bodies; in concrete clinical practices, business transactions, and state and EU regulations; as forms of speculative capital in the emergent market on personalized medicine; and in the hopes and dreams of the predominantly female consumers.

Concluding Remarks

In this book I have centered how three reproductive donations circulate in concrete local and global practices, in the cultural imagination, and in different mediated environments to become waste (actual waste or waste-in-the-making) and value (affective value, investment value, commercial value, etc.). Throughout the book I have offered a feminist approach to reproductive mobility, and I have chosen the term *global fluids* to embrace the ways in which three reproductive donations move across national boundaries and blur boundaries between what can be understood as gifts and commodities and what gets constructed as a consumable and a non-consumable object. While urine, eggs, and placenta come from women's reproductive bodies, they enter into vastly different circulations and value formations. When understood as global fluids, however, reproductive donations can be seen as being capable of changing more easily, not only with regard to their potential commodity state but also with regard to their entanglements with the world of finance, as things that are more readily convertible into compensation or investment potential.[5] As we have evidenced here, reproductive fluids encapsulate movement and transformability, gift-giving and economics.

Returning to the question of the cultural *politics* of reproduction: what is political about reproductive waste and value? In this concluding chapter, I have pointed to a cultural politics of reusability and extensibility as uniting all of the three case studies. When viewed from the perspectives offered by feminist cultural politics, the ways in which reproductive fluids come to matter as waste, products, brands, future cures, white beautiful skin, silky hair, or potential future children move beyond the specificity of a particular reproductive fluid. Here, global fluids come to constitute particular understandings of the reproductive body, including pharmaceutical and philanthropic bodies; rightful, informational, bland as well as exotic, ageless reproductive bodies; and entrepreneurial, neoliberal, regenerative, and ecological reproductive bodies. As demonstrated in these chapters, reproductive waste and value are cultural and also political. Reproductive waste and value transform not only female bodies but also our very understanding of what comes to constitute reproductive waste, including the ways that reproductive matter circulates in and out of different biopolitical regimes.

Notes

1. BioNews, "Students Sell Eggs to Pay Way through University," 25 November 2002, http://www.bionews.org.uk/page_11504.asp (retrieved August 2016).
2. In their publications, the Danish ethical council details what they see as moral dilemmas associated with assisted reproductive technologies. For more information consult the Danish ethical council website: http://www.etiskraad.dk/~/media/Etisk-Raad/Etiske-Temaer/Sundhedsvaesenet/Publikationer/2013-11-01-handel-aag-surrogatmoderskab-organer.pdf (retrieved August 2016).
3. For more comments about this specific episode, which took place at Poole Hospital in Dorset, United Kingdom, in 2007, read Sawer (2008).
4. Viking Genetics, "About VikingJersey," 2017, http://www.vikinggenetics.com/dairy/vikingjersey/about-vikingjersey (retrieved August 2017).
5. Dictionary.com, "Fluid," http://www.dictionary.com/browse/fluid (retrieved August 2016).

BIBLIOGRAPHY

Adams, V., M. Murphy, and A. E. Clarke. 2009. "Anticipation: Technoscience, Life, Affect, Temporality." *Subjectivity* 28: 246–65.

Adrian, S. W. 2016. "Nymaterielle teorier: Karen Barad." In *Kulturteorier og Kultursociologi,* edited by B. Schiermer, 77–100. Copenhagen: Hans Reitzels Forlag.

Adrian, S. W., and C. Kroløkke. 2018 "Passport to Parenthood: The Transnational Flow in Bodies and Gametes." *Nordic Journal of Feminist and Gender Research NORA.*

Ahmed, S. 2004. *The Cultural Politics of Emotion.* Edinburgh: Edinburgh University Press.

———. 2010. *The Promise of Happiness.* Durham, NC: Duke University Press.

Allen, R. 2016. "Is Egg Freezing Only for White Women?" *New York Times,* 21 May 2016. Retrieved May 2016 from http://mobile.nytimes.com/2016/05/22/opinion/is-egg-freezing-only-for-white-women.html?.

Almeling, R. 2009. "Gender and the Value of Bodily Goods: Commodification in Egg and Sperm Donation." *Law and Contemporary Problems* 72(3): 37–58.

———. 2011. *Sex Cells: The Medical Market for Eggs and Sperm.* Oakland: University of California Press.

Alter, C. 2016. "You Can Sell Your Poop for $13,000 a Year." *Time,* 30 January 2015. Retrieved January 2016 from http://time.com/3689384/you-can-sell-your-poop-for-13000-a-year/.

American Kidney Fund. 2016. "About Your Kidneys: What Do My Kidneys Do?" American Kidney Fund website. Retrieved October 2016 from http://www.kidneyfund.org/kidney-disease/about-your-kidneys.html#what_do_my_kidneys_do.

Appadurai, A. 1986. "Introduction: Commodities and the Politics of Value." In *The Social Life of Things: Commodities in Cultural Perspective,* edited by A. Appadurai, 3–63. Cambridge: Cambridge University Press.

———. 1996. *Modernity at Large: Cultural Dimensions of Globalization.* Minneapolis: University of Minnesota Press.

Arudou, D. 2013. "An Introduction to Japanese Society's Attitudes towards Race and Skin Color." In *The Melanin Millennium: Skin Color as 21st Century*

International Discourse, edited by R. E. Hall, 49–69. Dordrecht: Springer Science & Business Media.

Åsberg, C., and N. Lykke. 2010. "Feminist Technoscience Studies." *European Journal of Women's Studies* 17(4): 299–305.

Barad, K. 2003. "Posthumanist Performativity: Toward an Understanding of How Matter Comes to Matter." *Signs: Journal of Women in Culture and Society* 28(3): 801–31.

Bennett, T., and C. Healy. 2009. "Introduction." *Journal of Cultural Economy* 2(1–2): 3–10.

Berglund, S., and S. Lundin. 2012. "I Had to Leave: Making Sense of Buying a Kidney Abroad." In *The Body as Gift, Resource, and Commodity,* edited by M. Gunnorson and F. Svenaeus, 321–42. Södertörn: Södertörns Högskola.

Bergmann, S. 2011. "Reproductive Agency and Projects: Germans Searching for Egg Donation in Spain and the Czech Republic." *Reproductive BioMedicine Online* 23: 600–608.

Berlant, L. 2006. "Cruel Optimism." *Differences* 17(3): 20–26.

———. 2008. *The Female Complaint: The Unfinished Business of Sentimentality in American Culture.* Durham, NC: Duke University Press.

Bernardi, D. 2008. "Introduction: Race and Contemporary Hollywood Cinema." In *The Persistence of Whiteness: Race and Contemporary Hollywood Cinema,* edited by D. Bernardi, xv–xxvi. New York: Routledge.

Bestard, J. 2004. "Kinship and the New Genetics: The Changing Meaning of Biogenetic Substance." *Social Anthropology* 12(3): 253–63.

Bharadwaj, A. 2008. "Biosociality and Biocrossings: Encounters with Assisted Conception and Embryonic Stem Cells in India." In *Biosocialities, Genetics and the Social Sciences: Making Biologies and Identities,* edited by S. Gibbon and C. Novas, 98–116. Oxon: Routledge.

———. 2012. "The Other Mother: Supplementary Wombs and the Surrogate State in India." In *Reproductive Technologies as Global Form: Ethnographies of Knowledge, Practices, and Transnational Encounters,* edited by M. Knect, M. Klotz, and S. Beck, 139–60. New York: Campus Verlag.

Bharadwaj, A., and P. E. Glasner. 2009. *Local Cells, Global Science: The Rise of Embryonic Stem Cell Research in India.* New York: Routledge.

Birch, K. 2017. "Rethinking Value in the Bio-economy: Finance, Assetization, and the Management of Value." *Science, Technology, & Human Values* 42(3): 460–90.

Birch, K., and D. Tyfield. 2012. "Theorizing the Bioeconomy: Biovalue, Biocapital, Bioeconomics or . . . What?" *Science, Technology and Human Values* 38(3): 299–327.

Birrittieri, C. 2005. *What Every Woman Should Know about Fertility and Her Biological Clock.* Franklin Lakes, NJ: New Page Books.

Boyer, K. 2010. "Of Care and Commodities: Breast Milk and the New Politics of Mobile Biosubstances." *Progress in Human Geography* 34(1): 5–20.

Brown, N., A. Kraft, and P. Martin. 2006. "The Promissory Pasts of Blood Stem Cells." *Biosocieties* 1(3): 329–48.

Butler, J. 1993. *Bodies That Matter: On the Discursive Limits of "Sex."* New York: Routledge.

Callon, M. 1998. *The Laws of the Markets.* Oxford: Blackwell Publishers.

Carroll, K., and C. Kroløkke. 2017. "Freezing for Love: Enacting 'Responsible' Reproductive Citizenship through Egg Freezing." *Culture, Health & Sexuality. An International Journal for Research, Intervention and Care:* 1–14. Retrieved 12 October 2017 from Online First.

Casper, M. J., and A. E. Clarke. 1998. "Making the Pap Smear into the 'Right Tool' for the Job: Cervical Cancer Screening in the USA, circa 1940–95." *Social Studies of Science* 28(2): 255–90.

Cavanagh, S. 2010. *Queering Bathrooms: Gender, Sexuality, and the Hygienic Imagination.* Toronto: University of Toronto Press.

Clarke, A., L. Mamo, J. R. Fosket, J. R. Fishman, and J. K. Shim. 2010. *Biomedicalization: Technoscience, Health, and Illness in the U.S.* Durham, NC: Duke University Press.

Clarke, A. J. 2004. "Maternity and Materiality: Becoming a Mother in Consumer Culture." In *Consuming Motherhood,* edited by J. S. Taylor, L. L. Layne, and D. F. Wozniak, 55–71. New Brunswick, NJ: Rutgers University Press.

Cody, L. F. 2005. *Birthing the Nation: Sex, Science, and the Conception of Eighteenth-Century Britons.* Oxford: Oxford University Press.

Cohen, L. 2005. "Operability, Bioavailability, & Exception." In *Global Assemblages,* edited by A. Ong and S. Collier, 79–90. Oxford: Blackwell.

Colen, S. 1995. "'Like a Mother to Them': Stratified Reproduction and West Indian Childcare Workers and Employers in New York." In *Conceiving the New World Order: The Global Politics of Reproduction,* edited by F. D. Ginsburg and R. Rapp, 78–102. Oakland: University of California Press.

Conradsen, D. 2003. "Geographies of Care: Spaces, Practices, Experiences." *Social & Cultural Geography* 4(4): 451–54.

Cooper, M. 2008. *Life as Surplus: Biotechnology and Capitalism in the Neoliberal Era.* Seattle: Washington University Press.

Cooper, M., and C. Waldby. 2014 *Clinical Labor: Tissue donors and Research Subjects in the Bioeconomy.* Durham, NC: Duke University Press.

Copeman, J. 2009. "Introduction: Blood Donation, Bioeconomy, Culture." *Body & Society* 15(2): 1–28.

Council of Europe. 1997. "The Explanatory Report on the European Treaty Series—No. 164." Retrieved September 2017 from https://rm.coe.int/16800ccde5.

Curtis, A. 2010. "Giving 'Til It Hurts: Egg Donation and the Costs of Altruism." *Feminist Formations* 22(2): 80–100.

Daniels, C. R. 2006. *Exposing Men: The Science and Politics of Male Reproduction.* Oxford: Oxford University Press.

Daniels, C. R., and J. Golden. 2004. "Procreative Compounds: Popular Eugenics, Artificial Insemination and the Rise of the American Sperm Banking Industry." *Journal of Social History* 38(1): 5–27.

Danish Council on Ethics. 2012. "Udtalelse om compensation for aegdonation" (Opinion on Compensation for Egg Donation). Retrieved February 2016 from http://www.etiskraad.dk/da-dk/Nyhedsarkiv/2013/februar/~/media/bibliotek/udtalelser/2013/DER-Udtalelse-om-kompensation-for-aegdonation.pdf.

Danish Council on Ethics. 2013. "International handel med menneskelige æg, rugemoderskab og organer" (International trade with human eggs, surrogacy, and organs). Retrieved February 2016 from http://www.etiskraad.dk/etiske-temaer/sundhedsvaesenet/publikationer/handel-med-aeg-rugemoderskab-og-organer-redegoerelse-2013.

DasGupta, S, and S. Das Dasgupta. 2010. "Motherhood Jeopardized: Reproductive Technologies in Indian Communities." In *Conceiving the New World Order: The Global Politics of Reproduction*, edited by F. Ginsburg and R. Rapp, 78–103. Oakland: University of California Press.

Denbow, J. M. 2015. *Governed through Choice: Autonomy, Technology, and the Politics of Reproduction.* New York: New York University Press.

Devlin, L. 2014. "Why Do People Eat Placentas?" *BBC News*, 11 May 2014. Retrieved February 2015 from http://www.bbc.com/news/uk-england-27307476.

Dickenson, D. 2007. *Property in the Body: Feminist Perspectives.* Cambridge: Cambridge University Press.

———. 2009. *Body Shopping: Converting Body Parts to Profit.* Oxford: Oneworld Books.

Dickinson, E., K. A. Foss, and C. Kroløkke. 2016. "Empowering Disgust: Redefining Alternative Postpartum Placenta Practices." *Women's Studies in Communication* 40(1): 111–28.

"Do it for Denmark." 2013. Spies Travels, YouTube video. Retrieved September 2016 from: https://www.youtube.com/watch?v=vrO3TfJc9Qw

"Do it for Mom." 2015. Spies Travels, YouTube video. Retrieved September 2016 from: https://www.youtube.com/watch?v=B00grl3K01g

Douglas, M. (1966) 1984. *Purity and Danger: An Analysis of Concepts of Pollution and Taboo.* New York: Routledge.

———. 1990. "Foreword." In M. Mauss, *The Gift: The Form and Reason for Exchange in Archaic Societies.* Translated by W. Halls. London: Routledge.

Duden, B. 1993. *Disembodying Women: Perspectives on Pregnancy and the Unborn.* Cambridge: Harvard University Press.

Duggan, L. 2003. *The Twilight of Equality? Neoliberalism, Cultural Politics, and the Attack on Democracy.* Boston: Beacon Press.

Echlin, H. 2011. "Eating the Placenta: It Tastes like Squab!" Chowhound, 6 September 2011. Retrieved August 2016 from http://www.chowhound.com/food-news/90029/eating-the-placenta-it-tastes-like-squab/.

"Egg Donations in Ireland: New Beginnings Happen Every Day at Sims IVF." 2017. Sims IVF. Retrieved May 2017 from http://www.eggdonation.ie/_fileupload/NS1607%20EDE_web_brochure_v4.pdf.

Ericson, R., D. Barry, and A. Doyle. 2000. "The Moral Hazards of Neoliberalism: Lessons from the Private Insurance Industry." *Economy and Society* 29(4): 532–58.

Foss, S. 1984. "Women Priests in the Episcopal Church: A Cluster Analysis of Establishment Rhetoric." *Religious Communication Today* 7: 1–11.

Foss, K. A., S. K., Foss, and C. L. Griffin. 1999. *Feminist Rhetorical Theories.* Long Grove, IL: Waveland Press, Inc.

———. 2004. *Readings in Feminist Rhetorical Theory.* Long Grove, IL: Waveland Press, Inc.

Fox, R. C., and J. P. Swazey. 1992. *Spare Parts: Organ Replacement in American Society.* New York: Oxford University Press.

Franklin, S. 1997. *Embodied Progress: A Cultural Account of Assisted Conception.* London: Routledge.

———. 2001. "Biologization Revisited: Kinship Theory in the Context of the New Biologies." In *Relative Value: Reconfiguring Kinship Studies,* edited by S. Franklin and S. McKinnon, 302–25, Durham, NC: Duke University Press.

———. 2005. "Stem Cells R Us: Emergent Life Forms and the Global Biological." In *Global Assemblages: Technology, Politics and Ethics as Anthropological Problems,* edited by A. Ong and S. Collier, 59–78, Malden: Blackwell.

———. 2006. "Embryonic Economies: The Double Reproductive Value of Stem Cells. *BioSocieties* 1(1): 71–90.

———. 2007. *Dolly Mixtures: The Remaking of Genealogy.* Durham, NC: Duke University Press.

———. 2013. *Biological Relatives: IVF, Stem Cells, and the Future of Kinship.* Durham, NC: Duke University Press.

Franklin, S., C. Lury, and J. Stacey. 2000. *Global Nature, Global Culture.* Thousand Oaks, CA: Sage Publications.

Frow, J. 2003. "Invidious Distinctions: Waste, Difference, and Classy Stuff." In *Culture and Waste: The Creation and Destruction of Value,* edited by G. Hawkins and S. Muecke, 25–38, Lanham, MD: Rowman and Littlefield.

———. 1997. *Time and Commodity Culture: Essays in Theory and Postmodernity.* Oxford: Clarendon Press.

Gan, N. 2014. "Drinking Your Own Urine: The Unorthodox Chinese 'Miracle Cure.'" *South China Morning Post,* 2 July 2014. Retrieved October 2016 from http://www.scmp.com/news/china-insider/article/1544386/drinking-your-own-urine-unorthodox-chinese-miracle-cure.

Gelis, J. 1996. *History of Childbirth: Fertility, Pregnancy and Birth in Early Modern Europe.* Cambridge: Polity.

Glenn, E. N. 2008. "Yearning for Lightness: Transnational Circuits in the Marketing and Consumption of Skin Ligheners." *Gender and Society* 22(3): 281–302.

———. 2009. *Shades of Difference: Why Skin Color Matters.* Palo Alto: Stanford University Press.

Ginsburg, F. D., and R. Rapp (eds.). 1995. *Conceiving the New World Order: The Global Politics of Reproduction.* Berkeley: University of California Press.

Ginsburg F., and R. Rapp. 1991. "The Politics of Reproduction." *Annual Review of Anthropology* 20: 311–43.

"Global Fertility Services Market to Exceed USD 21 Billion by 2020, According to Technavio." 2016. Business Wire, 20 April 2016.

Gnoth, C., and S. Johnson. 2014. "Strips of Hope: Accuracy of Home Pregnancy Tests and New Developments." *Ceburtshilfe Frauenhelikd* 74(7): 661–69.

Goldblatt, H. 2000. "Forbidden Food: 'The Saturnicon' of Mo Yan." *World Literature Today* 74(3): 477–85.

Gunnarson, G., and F. Svenaeus (eds.). 2012. *Exchanging Organs, Tissues, and Cells in the 21st Century.* Södertörn: Södertörn Högskola.

Gupta, J., and A. Richters. 2008. "Embodied Subjects and Fragmented Objects: Women's Bodies, Assisted Reproduction Technologies and the Right to Self-Determination." *Bioethical Inquiry* 5(4): 239–49.

Gupta, J. A. 2006. "Towards Transnational Feminisms: Some Reflections and Concerns in Relation to the Globalization of Reproductive Technologies." *European Journal of Women's Studies* 13(1): 23–38.

Haraway, D. 1991. "The Promises of Monsters: A Regenerative Politics for Inapproriate/d Others." In *Cultural Studies,* edited by L. Grossberg, C. Nelson, P. Treichler, 295–337. New York: Routledge.

———. 1997. *Modest_Witness@Second_Millennium.FemaleMan_Meets_OncoMouse: Feminism and Technoscience.* New York: Routledge.

———. 2004. *The Haraway Reader.* New York: Routledge.

Green, S. G. 2015. "Ny kampagne: Få børn allerede mens du læser" (New campaign: Have children while you study). DR, 5 October 2015. Retrieved September 2016 from: https://www.dr.dk/levnu/parforhold/ny-kampagne-faa-boern-allerede-mens-du-laeser

Hawkins, G. 2003. "Down the Drain: Shit and the Politics of Disturbance." In *Culture and Waste: The Creation and Destruction of Value,* edited by G. Hawkins and S. Muecke, 39–52, Lanham, MD: Rowman and Littlefield.

———. 2011. "The Politics of Bottled Water: Assembling Bottled Water as Brand, Waste and Oil." In *Assembling Culture,* edited by T. Bennett and C. Healy, 177–89. London: Routledge.

Hawkins, G., and S. Muecke. 2003. "Introduction: Cultural Economics of Waste." In *Culture and Waste: The Creation and Destruction of Value,* edited by G. Hawkins and S. Muecke, ix–xvii, Lanham, MD: Rowman and Littlefield.

Hayden, S., and L. Hallstein. 2010. *Contemplating Maternity in an Era of Choice: Explorations into Discourses of Reproduction.* Lanham, MD: Lexington Books.

Hayles, K. N. 1999. *How We Became Posthuman: Virtual Bodies in Cybernetics, Literature and Informatics.* Chicago: The University of Chicago Press.

Hays, S. 1996. *The Cultural Contradictions of Motherhood.* New Haven, CT: Yale University Press.

Herring, C., V. M. Keith, and H. D. Horton (eds.). 2003. *Skin Deep: How Race and Complexion Matter in the "Color Blind" Era.* Chicago: Institute for Research on Race and Public Policy.

Hill, J. 2015. "Divorced Couple's Embryos Must Be Destroyed, US Judge Rules." BioNews, 23 November 2015. Retrieved August 2016 from http://www.bionews.org.uk/page_588452.asp.

Hillsman, P. 2016. "The Incredible Story of How Large Quantities of Nuns' Urine Made Fertility Drugs Possible." Raw Story, June 27. Retrieved October 2016 from https://www.rawstory.com/2016/06/the-incredible-story-of-how-large-quantities-of-nuns-urine-made-fertility-drugs-possible/.

Hochschild, A. 1979. "Emotion Work, Feeling Rules, and Social Structure." *American Journal of Sociology* 85(3): 551–75.

Hoeyer, K. 2013. *Exchanging Human Bodily Material: Rethinking Bodies and Markets.* New York: Springer.

Hogle, L. 1995. "Standardization across Non-Standard Domains: The Case of Organ Procurement." *Science, Technology, & Human Values* 20(4): 482–500.

Holliday, R., D. Bell, O. Cheung, M. Jones, and E. Probyn. 2015. "Brief Encounters: Assembling Cosmetic Surgery Tourism." *Social Science and Medicine* 124: 298–304.

Holmberg, T., N. Schwennesen, and A. Webster. 2011. "Bio-objects and the Bio-objectification Process." *Croatian Medical Journal* 52(6): 740–42.

Hunter, M. 2005. *Race, Gender, and the Politics of Skin Tone.* New York: Routledge.

———. 2007. "The Persistent Problem of Colorism: Skin Tone, Status, and Inequality." *Sociology Compass* 1(1): 237–54.

———. 2011. "Buying Racial Capital: Skin-Bleaching and Cosmetic Surgery in a Globalized World." *Journal of Pan African Studies* 4 (4): 142–64.

Hunter, M. L. 2002. "'If You're Light You're Alright': Light Skin Color as Social Capital for Women of Color." *Gender and Society* 16(2): 175–93.

Ingold, T. 1993. "Technology, Language, Intelligence: A Reconsideration of Basic Concepts." In *Language and Cognition in Human Evolution,* edited by K. R. Gibsen and T. Ingold, 449–72, Cambridge: Cambridge University Press.

Inhorn, M. C. 2010. "'Assisted' Motherhood in Global Dubai: Reproductive Tourists and Their Helpers." In *The Globalization of Motherhood: Deconstructions and Reconstructions of Biology and Care,* edited by J. M. Maher and W. Chavkin, 180–202, New York: Routledge.

———. 2011. "Globalization and Gametes: Reproductive 'Tourism,' Islamic Bioethics, and Middle Eastern Modernity." *Anthropology & Medicine* 18(1): 87–103.

———. 2015. *Cosmopolitan Conceptions: IVF Sojourns in Global Dubai.* Durham, NC: Duke University Press.

Inhorn, M. C., and P. Shrivastav. 2010. "Globalization and Reproductive Tourism in the United Arab Emirates." *Asia Pacific J Public Health* 22(3 Suppl): 68S–74S.

Intervet. 2016. "Same Time, Same Place: The Management Tool in Swine Reproduction." The Pig Site. Retrieved September 2016 from http://www.thepigsite.com/focus/contents/PG600%20061797.pdf.

Irigaray, L. 2007. *Je, Tu, Nous: Toward a Culture of Difference.* New York: Routledge.

Jackson, M. 2002. "Familiar and Foreign Bodies: A Phenomenological Exploration of the Human-Technology Interface." *Royal Anthropological Institute* 8: 333–46.

Jacobsen, E. 2004. "The Rhetoric of Food: Food as Nature, Commodity and Culture." In *The Politics of Food,* edited by M. E. Lien and B. Nerlich, 59–78, Oxford: Berg.

Jhally, S. 1989. "Advertising as Religion: The Dialectic of Technology and Magic." In *Cultural Politics in Contemporary America,* edited by I. Angus and S. Jhally. 217–29. New York: Routledge.

Jones, A. 2016. "Your Body Is a Goldmine (If You So Choose): Selling Body Parts for Cash." And Then We Saved. Retrieved January 2016 from http://andthenwesaved.com/selling-body-parts-for-cash/.

Jones, E., and M. A. Kay. 2003. "The Cultural Anthropology of the Placenta." In *The Manner Born: Birth Rites in Cross-Cultural Perspective,* edited by L. Dundes, 101–16. Lanham, MD: AltaMira Press.

Jordan, J. W. 2004. "The Rhetorical Limits of the 'Plastic Body.'" *Quarterly Journal of Speech* 90(3): 327–58.

Keating, P., and A. Cambriosio. 2003. *Biomedical Platforms: Realigning the Normal and the Pathological in Late-Twentieth-Century Medicine.* Cambridge, MA: The MIT Press.

Kelly, E. 2014. "New Mothers Defend Right to Eat Their Placentas after European Ruling." The Metro, 8 July 2014. Retrieved February 2015 from http://metro.co.uk/2014/07/08/new-mothers-defend-right-to-eat-their-placenta-after-european-ruling-4790013/.

Kietzer, L. 2012. "Three Times a Woman: A Gendered Economy of Stem Cell Innovation." eScholarship. Retrieved March 2015 from https://escholarship.org/dist/prd/content/qt70h7k694/qt70h7k694.pdf?t=mhint.

Kitzinger, S. 1979. *The Experience of Childbirth.* London: Penguin Books.

Kjær, B. 2015. "Derfor spiste vi vores moderkager." Livsstil.tv2.dk, 23 August 2013. Retrieved February 2015 from http://livsstil.tv2.dk/kropogsundhed/2013-08-23-derfor-spiste-vi-vores-moderkager.

Klotz, M., and S. Beck. 2012. *Reproductive Technologies as Global Form: Ethnographies of Knowledge, Practices, and Transnational Encounters.* Frankfurt: Campus Verlag.

Knaplund, K. S. 2004. "Postmortem Conception and a Father's Last Will." *Arizona Law Review* 46: 91–115.

Knecht, M., M. Klotz, and S. Beck. 2012. *Reproductive Technologies as Global Form: Ethnographies of Knowledge, Practices, and Transnational Encounters.* Frankfurt and Chicago: Campus.

Knudsen, I. H., and M. Frederiksen. 2015. *Ethnographies of Grey Zones in Eastern Europe: Relations, Borders, and Invisibilities.* New York: Anthem Press.

Konrad, M. 2000. "Ova Donation and Symbols of Substance: Some Variations on the Theme of Sex, Gender and the Partible Body." *Journal of the Royal Anthropological Institute (N.S.)* 4: 643–67.

———. 2005. *Nameless Relations: Anonymity, Melanesia and Reproductive Gift Exchange between British Ova Donors and Recipients.* Oxford: Berghahn Books.

Kopytoff, I. 1986. "The Cultural Biography of Things: Commoditization as Process." In *The Social Life of Things,* edited by A. Appadurai, 64–91. Cambridge: Cambridge University Press.

Kristeva, J. 1982. *Powers of Horror: An Essay on Abjection.* New York: European Perspectives, Columbia University Press.

Kroløkke, C. 2009. "Click a Donor: Viking Masculinity on the Line." *Journal of Consumer Culture* 9(1): 7–30.

———. 2011. "Biotourist Performances: Doing Parenting during the Ultrasound." *Text and Performance Quarterly* 31(1): 15–36.

———. 2012. "From India with Love: Troublesome Citizens of Fertility Travel." *Cultural Politics* 8(2): 307–25.

———. 2014. "West Is Best: Affective Assemblages and Spanish Oöcytes." *European Journal of Women's Studies* 21(1): 57–71.

———. 2015a. "Have Eggs,Will Travel: The Ethics of Global Egg Donation." *Journal of Somatechnics: Special Issue on Medical Travel and Bioethics* 5(1): 12–31.

———. 2015b. "The Golden Egg: The Business of Making Motherhood through Egg Donation." In *The Motherhood Business: Consumption, Communication and Privilege,* edited by A. Demo, J. Borda, and C. Kroløkke, 28–51, Tuscaloosa: University of Alabama Press.

———. 2016a. "Jetlagged and Bloated: Egg Provider Tourism and Transformations." In *Global Bodies in Grey Zone: Health, Hope, and Biotechnology,* edited by S. Lundin, C. Kroløkke, M. N. Petersen, E. Muller, 75–90. Stellenbosch: SUNMeDIA.

———. 2016b. "ART in the Sun: Assembling Fertility Tourism in the Caribbean." In *Critical Kinship: Kinship Transformed,* edited by C. Kroløkke, L. Myong, S. W. Adrian, and T. Tjørnhøj-Thomsen, 149–66. London: Rowman and Littlefield.

Kroløkke, C., E. Dickinson, and K. Foss. 2016. "The Placenta Economy. From Trashed to Treasured Bio-Products." *European Journal of Women's Studies,* iFirst: 1–15.

Kroløkke, C., K. Foss, and S. Pant. 2012. "Fertility Travel: The Commodification of Human Reproduction." *Cultural Politics* 8(2): 273–82.

Kroløkke, C., and S. Pant. 2012, "'I Only Need Her Uterus': Neoliberal Discourses on Transnational Surrogacy." *NORA—Nordic Journal of Feminist and Gender Research* 20(4): 233–48.

Kroløkke, C., and M. Nebeling Petersen. 2017. "Keeping It in the Family: Debating the Bio-intimacy of Uterine Transplants and Commercial Surrogacy." In *Bioethics beyond Altruism: Donating and Transforming Human Biological Materials,* edited by R. Shaw, 189–213. New York: Palgrave Macmillan.

Lakoff, G., and M. Johnson. 1980. *Metaphors We Live By.* Chicago: University of Chicago Press.

Landecker, H. 2007. *Cultural Life: How Cells Became Technologies.* Cambridge: Harvard University Press.

Largey, G. P., and D. R. Watson. 1972. "The Sociology of Odours." *American Journal of Sociology* 77(6): 1021–34.

Lash, S., and C. Lury. 2007. *Global Culture Industry: The Mediation of Things.* Cambridge: Polity.

Lay, M. M., L. J. Gurak, C. Gravon, and C. Myntti (eds.). 2000. *Body Talk: Rhetoric, Technology, Reproduction.* Madison: University of Wisconsin Press.

Layne, L. L. 2009. "The Home Pregnancy Test: A Feminist Technology?" *Women's Studies Quarterly* 37(1–2): 61–79.

Lemke, T. 2001. "The Birth of Bio-Politics: Michel Foucault's Lecture at the Collége de France on Neo-liberal Governmentality." *Economy and Society* 30(2): 190–207.

Lie, M. 2012. "Reproductive Images: The Autonomous Cell." *Science as Culture,* iFirst: 1–22.

Lie, M., and N. Lykke. 2017. "Editorial Introduction: Assisted Reproduction across Borders; Feminist Perspectives on Normalizations, Disruptions and Transmissions." In *Assisted Reproduction across Borders: Feminist Perspectives on Normalizations, Disruptions and Transmissions,* edited by M. Lie and N. Lykke, 1–21. New York: Routledge.

Long, E. C. 1963. "The Placenta in Lore and Legend." *Bulletin of the Medical Library Association* 51(2): 233–41.

Longhurst, R. 2001. *Bodies: Exploring Fluid Boundaries.* London: Routledge.

Lunenfeld, B. 2004. "Historical Perspectives in Gonadotrophin Therapy." *Human Reproduction Update* 10(6): 453–67.

Lury, C. 2009. "Brand as Assemblage." *Journal of Consumer Cultural Economy* 2(1–2): 67–82.

———. 2011. *Consumer Culture.* New Brunswick, NJ: Rutgers University Press.

Malmqvist, E. 2012. "Trading Hair, Trading Cadaver Tissue: On the Ethics of Commodifying Bodily Sacrifices and Gifts." In *Exchanging Organs, Tissues, and Cells in the 21st Century,* edited by M. Gunnarson and F. Svenaeus, 296–320, Södertörn: Södertörn Högskola.

Mamo, L. 2007. *Queering Reproduction: Achieving Pregnancy in the Age of Technoscience.* Durham, NC: Duke University Press.

Marcus, G. 1999. "What Is at Stake—and Is Not—In the Idea and Practice of Multi-sited Ethnography." *Canberra Anthropology, The Asia Pacific Journal of Anthropology* 22(2): 6–14.

Marcus, G., and E. Saka. 2006. "Assemblage." *Theory, Culture and Society* 23(2–3): 101–16.

Markens, S. 2007. *Surrogate Motherhood and the Politics of Reproduction.* Berkeley: University of California Press.

Martin, E. 1987. *The Woman in the Body: A Cultural Analysis of Reproduction.* Boston: Beacon.

———. 1991. "The Egg and the Sperm: How Science Has Constructed a Romance Based on Stereotypical Male-Female Roles." *Signs: Journal of Women in Culture and Society* 16(3): 485–501.

———. 1994. *Flexible Bodies: The Role of Immunity in American Culture from the Days of Polio to the Age of AIDS.* Boston: Beacon Press.

———. 1998. "Fluid Bodies, Managed Nature." In *Remaking Reality: Nature at the Millenium,* edited by B. Braun and N. Castree, 64–83. New York: Routledge.

———. 2006. "The Pharmaceutical Person." *BioSocieties* 1(3): 273–87.

Mauss, M. (1950) 1990. *The Gift: The Form and Reason for Exchange in Archaic Societies.* Translated by W. Halls. Foreword by M. Douglas. London: Routledge.

Maxted, A. 2014. "Meet the Mothers Who Want to Eat Their Placentas." *The Telegraph*, August 5. Retrieved February 2015 from http://www.telegraph.co.uk/women/womens-health/11012491/Meet-the-mothers-who-eat-their-placentas.html.

Mikkelsen, A. L. 2015. "Efterbyrder løfter Elbjergs bundlinje." *Effektivt Landbrug*: 8–9.

Mol, A. M. 2002. *The Body Multiple: Ontology in Medical Practice*. Durham, NC: Duke University Press.

Mol, A., and J. Law. 1994. "Regions, Networks and Fluids: Anaemia and Social Topology." *Social Studies of Science* 24(4): 641–71.

Melhuus, M. 2012. *Problems of Conception: Issues of Law, Biotechnology, Individuals, and Kinship*. Oxford: Berghahn Books.

Morgan, C. J. 2016. "Five Ways to Make Cash Selling Your Body to Science." CJ's Blog, 16 November 2015. Retrieved January 2016 from http://www.klbjfm.com/blogs/cjs-blog/five-ways-make-cash-selling-your-body-science.

Morgan, L. M. 2013. "The Potentiality Principle from Aristotle to Abortion." *Current Anthropology* 54(S7): S15–S25.

Morse, M. 1990. "An Ontology of Everyday Distraction." In *Logics of Television: Essays in Cultural Criticism*, edited by P. Mellemcamp, 193–222, Bloomington: Indiana University Press.

Moser, W. 2002. "The Acculturation of Waste." In *Waste-Site Stories: The Recycling of Memory*, edited by B. Neville and J. Villeneuve, 85–106, Albany: State University of New York Press.

Mølgaard, M. 2015. "Ægge-kampagne skal få unge til at få børn: Her er kvindernes geniale svar" (Egg campaign is aiming to have young women have children: Here are the women's genious responses). *BT*, 8 October 2015. https://www.bt.dk/danmark/aegge-kampagne-skal-faa-unge-til-at-faa-boern-her-er-kvindernes-geniale-svar.

Myddleton, W. W. 1959. "Modern Trends in Cosmetic Formulation." *Journal of the Society of Cosmetic Chemists*: 192–204.

Nadesan, M. J., and A. Trethewey. 2000. "Performing the Enterprising Subject: Gendered Strategies for Success(?)." *Text and Performance Quarterly* 20(3): 223–30.

Nahman, M. 2006. "Materializing Israeliness: Difference and Mixture in Transnational Ova Donation." *Science as Culture* 15(3): 199–213.

———. 2008. "Nodes of Desire: Romanian Egg Sellers, 'Dignity' and Feminist Alliances in Transnational Ova Exchange." *European Journal of Women's Studies* 15(2): 65–82.

———. 2011. "Reverse Traffic: Intersecting Inequalities in Human Egg Donation." *Reproductive Biomedicine Online* 23(5): 626–33.

———. 2012. "Making Interferences: The Cultural Politics of Transnational Ova 'Donation.'" In *Reproductive Technologies as Global Form: Ethnographies of Knowledge, Practices, and Transnational Encounters*, edited by M. Knect, M. Klotz, and S. Beck, 305–30, Frankfurt: Campus Verlag.

———. 2013. *Extractions: An Ethnography of Reproductive Tourism*. Hampshire: Palgrave Macmillan.

Nebeling, M., C. Kroløkke, and L. Myong. 2016. "Dad and Daddy Assemblages: Norwegian Homo- and Repro-Nationalism." *GLQ—A Journal of Gay and Lesbian Studies* 23(1): 83–112.

Newman, C. E., M. Bonar, H. S. Greville, S. C. Thompson, D. Bessarab, and S. C. Kippax. 2007. "'Everything Is Okay': The Influence of Neoliberal Discourse on the Reported Experiences of Aboriginal People in Western Australia Who Are HIV-Positive." *Culture, Health & Sexuality* 9(6): 571–84.

Nielsen, C. 2014. "Dansk tyresæd er på vej til Thailand" (Danish bull sperm is on its way to Thailand). DR, 29 January 2014. Retrieved February 2014 from http://www.dr.dk/nyheder/regionale/oestjylland/dansk-tyresaed-er-paa-vej-til-thailand.

Novas, C. 2006. "The Political Economy of Hope: Patients' Organizations, Science and Biovalue." *BioSocieties* 1: 289–305.

Ong, A., and S. Collier, eds. 2005. *Global Assemblages: Technology, Politics, and Ethics as Anthropological Problems.* Oxford: Blackwell.

Orobitg, G., and C. Salazar. 2005. "The Gift of Motherhood: Egg Donation in a Barcelona Infertility Clinic." *Ethnos* 70(1): 31–52.

Oudshoorn, N. 1994. *Beyond the Natural Body: An Archeology of Sex Hormones.* London: Routledge.

Palmer, J. 2015. "Checking the Placenta." Pregnancy.com, 25 June 2015. Retrieved August 2016 from http://www.pregnancy.com.au/birth-choices/birth-information/labour-third-stage/checking-the-placenta.shtml.

Pande, A. 2009. "'It May Be Her Eggs but It's My Blood': Surrogates and Everyday Forms of Kinship in India." *Qualitative Sociology* 32: 379–97.

Parr, H. 2003. "Medical Geography: Care and Caring." *Progress in Human Geography* 27(2): 212–21.

Parry, B. 2007. "Entangled Exchange: Reconceptualising the Characterization and Practice of Bodily Commodification." *Geoforum* 39: 1133–44.

Passariello, P. 1994. "Sacred Waste: Human Body Parts as Universal Sacraments." *American Journal of Semiotics* 11(1–2): 109–27.

Pelley, L. 2016. "Placenta Pills: A Growing Trend, but Some Warn of Possible Risks." *The Star*, 25 January 2016. Retrieved August 2016 from https://thestar.com/life/health_wellness/2016/01/25/placenta-pills-a-growing-trend-but-some-warn-of-possible-risks.html.

Petchesky, R. P. 1995. "The Body as Property: A Feminist Re-vision." In *Conceiving the New World Order: The Global Politics of Reproduction,* edited by F. D. Ginsburg and R. Rapp, 387–406, Oakland: University of California Press.

Phillips, A. 2013. *Our Bodies: Whose Property?* Princeton, NJ: Princeton University Press.

Pink, S. 2009. *Doing Sensory Ethnography.* New York: SAGE Publications.

Pollock, A. 2003. "Complicating Power in High-Tech Reproduction: Narratives of Anonymous Paid Egg Donors." *Journal of Medical Humanities* 24(3–4): 241–63.

Pollock, D. 1999. *Telling Bodies Performing Birth.* New York: Columbia University Press.

Puar, J. 2007. *Terrorist Assemblage: Homonationalism in Queer Times.* Durham, NC: Duke University Press.

Puar, J. K. 2009. "Prognosis Time: Towards a Geopolitics of Affect, Debility and Capacity." *Women & Performance: A Journal of Feminist Theory* 19(2): 161–72.

Radin M. J. 1996. *Contested Commodities.* Cambridge: Harvard University Press.

Rajan, K. S. 2007. *Biocapital: The Constitution of Postgenomic Life.* Durham, NC: Duke University Press.

———. 2017. *Pharmocracy: Value, Politics, and Knowledge in Global Biomedicine.* Durham, NC: Duke University Press.

Raymond, J. 1993. *Women as Wombs: Reproductive Technologies and the Battle over Women's Freedom.* San Francisco: HarperSanFrancisco.

Roberts, E. F. S. 2012. *God's Laboratory: Assisted Reproduction in the Andes.* Oakland: University of California Press.

———. 2015. "Bio-Ethnography: A Collaborative, Methodological Experiment in Mexico City." *Somatosphere,* February 26. Retrieved October 2017 from http://somatosphere.net/2015/02/bio-ethnography.html.

Roberts, E. F. S. and N. Scheper-Hughes. 2011. "Introduction: Medical Migrations." *Body & Society* 17(2–3): 1–30.

Rose, N. 1999. *Powers of Freedom: Reframing Political Thought.* Cambridge: Cambridge University Press.

———. 2007. *The Politics of Life Itself: Biomedicine, Power, and Subjectivity in the Twenty-First Century.* Princeton, NJ: Princeton University Press.

Russell, C. 2015. "The Race Idea in Reproductive Technologies: Beyond Epistemic Scientism and Technological Mastery." *Journal of Bioethical Inquiry* 12(4): 601–12.

Santoro, P. 2011. "Liminal Biopolitics: Towards a Political Anthropology of the Umbilical Cord and the Placenta." *Body & Society* 17(1): 73–93.

Sauerwein, K. 2014. "Mom Smuggles Placenta after Hospital Refuses to Release It." Babycenter blog, 4 September 2014. Retrieved September 2014 from http://blogs.babycenter.com/mom_stories/09042014-mom-smuggles-placenta-eat-placenta/.

Sawer, P. 2008. "NHS Hospital Sells Placentas for Cosmetic Use." *The Telegraph,* 17 May 2008. Retrieved May 2014 from http://www.telegraph.co.uk/news/1973229/NHS-hospital-sells-placentas-for-cosmetic-use.html.

Sawicki, J. 1999. "Disciplining Mothers: Feminism and the New Reproductive Technologies." In *Feminist Theory and the Body: A Reader,* edited by J. Price and M. Shildrick, 190–202. Edinburgh: Edinburgh University Press.

Scheper-Hughes, N. 2000. "The Global Traffic in Human Organs." *Current Anthropology* 41(2). Retrieved April 2014 from http://www.jstor.org/discover/10.1086/300123?uid=3737880&uid=2129&uid=2&uid=70&uid=4&sid=21103941073057.

———. 2001. "Bodies for Sale—Whole or in Parts." *Body & Society* 7(2): 1–8.

———. 2005. "Bodies for Sale—Whole or in Parts." In *Commodifying Bodies,* edited by N. Scheper-Hughes and L. Wacquant, 1–8. London: Sage.

———. 2011. "Mr Tati's Holiday and Joao's Safari—Seeing the World through Transplant Tourism." *Body & Society* 17(2–3): 55–92.

———. 2015. "(IM)MOBILITY: Mobility For Whom?" *Roots & Routes: Research on Visual Culture* 5(20). Retrieved October 2016 from http://www.roots-routes.org/immobilitymobility-for-whomnancy-scheper-hughes-comments/.

Seigel, M. 2014. *The Rhetoric of Pregnancy.* Chicago: University of Chicago Press.

Shail, A. 2007. "'Although a Woman's Article': Menstruant Economics and Creative Waste." *Body & Society* 13(4): 77–96.

Shenfield, F., J. de Mouzon, G. Pennings, A. P. Ferraretti, A. Nyboe Andersen, G. de Wert, and V. Grossens. 2010. "The ESHRE Taskforce on Cross Border Reproductive Care in Six European Countries." *Human Reproduction.* 23: 2182–84.

Sharp, L. 2000. "The Commodification of the Body and Its Parts." *Annual Review of Anthropology* 29: 287–328.

Shaw, R. 2008. "Rethinking Reproductive Gifts as Body Projects." *Sociology* 42(1): 11–28.

Sheller, M., and J. Urry, eds. 2004. *Tourism Mobilities: Places to Stay, Places in Play.* London: Routledge.

———. 2006. "The New Mobilities Paradigm." *Environment and Planning A* 38: 207–26.

Shildrick, M. 1997. *Leaky Bodies and Boundaries: Feminism, Postmodernism and (Bio)Ethics.* New York: Routledge.

———. 2008. "The Critical Turn in Feminist Bioethics: The Case of Heart Transplantations." *Journal of Feminist Approaches to Bioethics* 1(1): 28–47.

Shrief, L. 2015. "PRESS RELEASE—IPEN Placenta Specialists and Food Hygiene Inspections." IPEN, 20 March 2015. Retrieved August 2016 from http://www.placentanetwork.com/press-release-ipen-placenta-specialists-and-food-hygiene-inspections-190315/.

———. 2015. "What about the Placenta? Why and How Thousands of Women Are Consuming Their Own Placentas." Toddle About Blog, 13 October 2015. Retrieved September 2016 from https://www.toddleabout.co.uk/blog/what-about-the-placenta-why-and-how-thousands-of-women-are-consuming-their-own-placentas/.

Skene, L. 2012. "Proprietary Interests in Human Bodily Material: Yearworth, Recent Australian Cases on Stored Semen and Their Implications." *Medical Law Review* 20(2): 227–45. doi:10.1093/medlaw/fws001.

Smith, D. 2015. "Watch Mum Drink Her Own PLACENTA in a Smoothie as She Bids to Boost Health after Giving Birth." *Mirror,* 26 February 2015. Retrieved April 2015 from http://www.mirror.co.uk/news/uk-news/watch-mum-drink-placenta-smoothie-5234159.

Smith, N. 1998. "Nature at the Millenium: Production and Re-enchantment." In *Remaking Reality: Nature at the Millenium,* edited by B. Braun and N. Castree, 271–85. New York: Routledge.

Spar, D. 2006. *The Baby Business: How Money, Science, and Politics Drive the Commerce of Conception.* Cambridge: Harvard Business Review Press.

Staff, K. 2016. "Pregnant Woman Wins Right to Her Placenta." Kare 11, 1 June 2016. Retrieved July 2016 from http://www.kare11.com/news/nation-now/pregnant-mississippi-woman-wins-right-to-her-placenta/226220557.

Stearn, C. A. 1999. "Breastfeeding and the Good Maternal Body." *Gender & Society* 13(3): 308–25.

Strasser, S. 1999. *Waste and Want: A Social History of Trash.* New York: Metropolitan.

Strathern, M. 1988. *The Gender of the Gift: Problems with Women and Problems with Society in Melanesia.* Oakland: University of California Press.

———. 1991. *Partial Connections.* Lanham, MD: Rowman and Littlefield.

———. 1992. *After Nature: English Kinship in the Late Twentieth Century.* Cambridge: Cambridge University Press.

———. 1999. *Property, Substance, and Effect: Anthropological Essays on Persons and Things.* London: Athlone.

Svendsen, M. N. 2014. "Selective Reproduction: Social and Temporal Imaginaries for Negotiating the Value of Life in Human and Animal Neonates." *Medical Anthropology Quarterly* 29(2): 178–95.

Tausk, M. 1975. *Pharmacology of Hormones.* Uppsala: Scientia Bokförlag.

Taussig K. S., K. Hoeyer, and S. Helmreich. 2013. "The Anthropology of Potentiality in Biomedicine: An Introduction to Supplement 7." *Current Anthropology* 54(S7): S3–S14.

Thompson, C. 2005. *Making Parents: The Ontological Choreography of Reproductive Technologies.* Cambridge: The MIT Press.

———. 2011. "Medical Migrations Afterword: Science as a Vacation?" *Body & Society* 17(2–3): 205–13.

———. 2013. *Good Science: The Ethical Choreography of Stem Cell Research.* Cambridge, MA: The MIT Press.

Thomsen, S. 2016. "Cryos vil lokke danske donorer til ægbank I udlandet" (Cryos wants to lure Danish donors to egg banks abroad). *Politiken,* 18 May 2016. Retrieved June 2016 from http://politiken.dk/forbrugogliv/sundhedogmotion/ECE3210852/cryos-vil-lokke-danske-donorer-til-aegbank-i-udlandet/.

Titmuss, R. M. 1970. *The Gift Relationship: From Human Blood to Social Policy.* London: Allan & Unwin.

Tober, D. 2001. "Semen as Gift, Semen as Goods: Reproductive Workers and the Market in Altruism." *Body & Society* 7: 137–60.

Toft, J. H. 2015. "Sæd, reagensglas og hormoner: Barnløshed er en milliardindustri i Danmark" (Seeds, test tubes, and hormones: Childlessness is a billion-dollar industry in Denmark). *Finans,* 25 December 2015. Retrieved September 2017 from http://finans.dk/finans/erhverv/ECE8308663/S%C3%A6d-reagensglas-og-hormoner-Barnl%C3%B8shed-er-en-milliardindustri-i-Danmark/?ctxref=ext.

Trommelen, J. 2013. "Zwangere vrouwen misleid door farmaceutisch bedrijf" (Pregnant women misled by pharmaceutical company). *de Volkskrant,* 27 May 2013. Retrieved January 2016 from http://www.volkskrant.nl/

vk/nl/2686/Binnenland/article/detail/3447753/2013/05/27/Farmaceutisch-bedrijf-misleidde-zwangeren.dhtml.

Umemura, M., and S. Slater. 2017. "Reaching for Global in the Japanese Cosmetics Industry, 1915 to 2015: The Case of Shiseido." *Business History* 59(6): 877–903.

Urry, J. 2000. *Sociology beyond Societies: Mobilities for the Twenty-First Century.* New York: Routledge.

Valentine, K. 2005. "Citizenship, Identity, Blood Donation." *Body & Society* 11(2): 113–28.

van de Wiel, L. 2015. "Freezing in Anticipation: Eggs for Later." *Women's Studies International Forum* 53 (November–December): 119–28.

———. 2016. "Cellular Origins: A Visual Analysis of Time-Lapse Embryo Imaging." In *Assisted Reproduction across Borders: Feminist Perspectives on Normalizations, Disruptions and Transmissions,* edited by M. Lie and N. Lykke, 288–301. New York: Routledge.

Vora, K. 2015. *Life Support: Biocapital and the New History of Outsourced Labor.* Minneapolis: University of Minnesota Press.

Wahlberg, A. 2018. *Good Quality: The Routinization of Sperm Banking in China.* Berkeley: University of California Press.

Waldby, C. 2000. *The Visible Human Project: Informatic Bodies and Posthuman Medicine.* London: Routledge.

———. 2006a. "Feminist Technoscience: Intimacy, Embodiment and Abjection in Science Studies." *Science Studies* 19(2): 3–5.

———. 2006b. "Umbilical Cord Blood: From Social Gift to Venture Capital." *Biosocieties* 1(1): 55–70.

———. 2010. "From Reproductive Work to Regenerative Labour: The Female Body and the Stem Cell Industries." *Feminist Theory* 11(1): 3–22.

———. 2014. "'Banking Time': Egg Freezing and the Negotiation of Future Fertility." *Culture, Health & Sexuality* 17(4): 470–82.

Waldby, C., and M. Cooper. 2008. "The Biopolitics of Reproduction: Post-Fordist Biotechnology and Women's Clinical Labour." *Australian Feminist Studies* 23(55): 57–73.

Waldby, C., and R. Mitchell. 2006. *Tissue Economies: Blood, Organs, and Cell Lines in Late Capitalism.* Durham, NC: Duke University Press.

Walkerdine, V., and P. Bansel. 2010. "Neoliberalism, Psychology and the Subject of Work." University of Sussex website. Retrieved March 2012 from www.sussex.ac.uk/cheer/documents/walkerdine.

Waskul, D. D., and P. Vannini. 2008. "Smell, Odor, and Somatic Work: Sense-Making and Sensory Management." *Social Psychology Quarterly* 71(1): 53–71.

Whippman, R. 2016. "Should I Defrost My Freezer Boys?" *The Guardian,* 28 May 2016. Retrieved May 2016 from http://www.theguardian.com/lifeandstyle/2016/may/28/ivf-frozen-embryos-pregnancy-ruth-whippman?CMP=fb_gu.

Zehr, M. 2017. "HCG Pregnyl & Weight Loss." Livestrong.com, 18 July 2017. Retrieved January 2016 from http://www.livestrong.com/article/320916-hcg-pregnyl-weight-loss/.

INDEX

A
abjection theory, 66
abortion, 7
agency, 26–27
Akzo Pharma, 16
alienation, 157
altruism, 153
  culture and, 4
  MvM and, 54, 55, 62, 76
  oocytes and, 88, 89, 141, 158
  philanthropic body and, 142
animals. *See* human-animal crossings
Aspen Oss, 77n8
  MvM and, 52, 54, 59
assemblage ethnography
  analytical and empirical tracking strategy for, 8, 9
  bio-ethnography and, 8
  bottled water campaigns and, 9
  empirical material in, 9–10, 14–15
  of oocytes, 81–83
  placentas and, 10
  of urine donation, 10

B
Barad, Karen, 31
Barbados, 84, 90, 104, 108n6, 159
  IVF holidays in, 8
  oocyte providers in, 82–83
Beyond the Natural Body: An Archeology of Sex Hormones (Oudshoorn), 55
bioart, 115, 128–29
biobanking, 130–31
biocapital, 37
  placenta and, 130
bio-crossings, 42–43
bio-ethnography, 8
bio-objectification, 34
biopower, 35
biovalue, 18
  global politics and, 39
  Waldby on, 38–39
bland reproductive bodies, 98–100
blood, 54, 55, 132
  kinship and, 70
  price of, plasma, 1
  urine donation compared to, 56–57, 60, 63
The Body Multiple: Ontology in Medical Practice (Mol), 30–31
breast milk, 74
  price of, 1
  urine donation and, 60

C
cadaver, 1
cannibalism, 119–20
class, 144
  whiteness and, 125–26, 128
colorism, 127
commodity framework, 90
  commodity situation in, 145–46
  as cultural, 141
  entrepreneurial body and, 142
  in feminist scholarship, 18

late-modern capitalism and, 143
for placentas, 17
reusability and extensibility and, 148
sperm donation in, 144–45, 147
transnational feminists on, 146
Copenhagen campaign. *See* Have You Counted Your Eggs Today?
cultural paths, 15

D

Denmark, 10, 14, 152
assisted reproduction law in, 11, 19n7
branding of reproductive matter in, 161–62
child support in, 12
cross-border fertility treatments and, 12, 16–17
Do It for Denmark and Do It for Mom campaign in, 22, 27–31
double donation in, 11
fertility problem in, 27
Have You Counted Your Eggs Today? campaign in, 22–24, 26
immigrants in, 12
IVF in, 11–12
placenta in clinical practices of, 115, 116, 118, 158
porcine placentas from, 5, 11, 17, 21, 43, 111–12, 117, 126–27, 136n6, 136n8, 159–60
race in reproduction campaigns in, 27
welfare state of, 11–12, 163
disciplined porous body, 74
flexibility and, 75
responsibility and, 76
disentanglement, 153
informed consent as, 151
regenerative labor as, 156
distributive value, of oocytes, 105–6
Do It for Denmark and Do It for Mom campaign, 22
activity in, 29
affect in, 28
naturalization in, 31
technology in, 30
wetness in, 27, 28, 29, 31
double donation, 11

E

egg freezing, 51n3, 83, 104–5, 162
babies and, 93–94
biocapital and, 37
cost of, 108n4
gender equality and, 87, 152–53
heterosexuality and, 106, 152–53
as investment, 85–87, 97
in Japan, 10, 14
laws in Denmark on, 11, 19n7
optimization and, 5
plasticity and, 86
reproductive value of, 106–7, 163
scarcity and, 85–86, 88
seminar for, 82
in United Kingdom, 10
in United States, 10, 14
waste and, 85
empowerment, 160
oocyte providers and, 100, 103, 105
placenta consumption and, 120, 127–28, 132–33, 154
entanglements, 15–16, 21, 49, 74, 159
disentanglement and, 151, 153, 156
global and local, 44, 160, 161
of oocytes, 91
of urine donation, 60
of waste and value, 38
entrepreneurial body, 25, 158
commodity framework and, 142
in feminist rhetorical and communication analysis, 23, 25, 26–27
gifting and, 155
neoliberalism and, 155–56
entrepreneurial value, 105–7
European Union
Convention on Human Rights and Biomedicine in, 13
novel food in, 132–33, 137n19
placenta in, 112, 132–33, 137n19

transnational markets and, 5
See also Denmark; Spain; United Kingdom
exotic bodies, 86–87, 101–3

F

feces, 35
femininity
gift and commodity framework and pan-femininity, 92–93
oocytes and globalized, 89, 92–93, 103, 107
regenerative labor and, 157–58
feminist affect and materialist analyses, 27, 32
activity in, 29
emotionality of texts and, 28
fertility coordinators and, 28–29
materialism in, 29–31
oocyte donation in, 33, 93–94
placenta consumption in, 33
practices in, 30–31
re-naturalization in, 31, 33
technology and, 30
See also Do It for Denmark and Do It for Mom campaign
feminist cultural analysis, 7, 22, 31, 50
assemblage ethnography and, 8
global in, 160
kin relations in, 32
oocytes in, 81
physical matter in, 32
placentas in, 113
of pregnancy test, 64
of urine, 3
See also feminist affect and materialist analyses; feminist rhetorical and communication analysis
feminist cultural politics, 7, 18–19
reusability and extensibility in, 140, 141, 159, 163–65
welfare state and, 163–64
feminist rhetorical and communication analysis, 32
birth stories in, 24
communication in, 23
entrepreneurial body in, 23, 25, 26–27
gendered practices in, 23
Have You Counted Your Eggs Today? campaign in, 22–24, 26
metaphors in, 24–25
of MvM, 61
neoliberal body in, 23–24, 26–27
philanthropic body in, 23, 26–27
placenta in, 118
feminist scholarship, 2–3
commodification in, 18
transnational feminists in, 146
fertilizer, 53
Findley v. Lee, 150–51

G

gendered practices
in feminist rhetorical and communication analysis, 23
menstruation and hierarchy in, 7
ordering of, 7
gender equality, 87, 152–53
gift and commodity framework, 6–7, 37, 83, 141
consumer choice in, 91, 92
emotional rewards in, 89–90
entrepreneurial body and, 155
neoliberalism and, 4
for oocytes, 88–93
pan-femininity in, 92–93
philanthropic body and, 142
reproductive quality and, 88–89
as social, 143
somatic work in, 90
urine donation and, 48–49, 59
See also commodity framework
gift market
gray thinking and, 141
IVF in, 145
objectification in, 149
philanthropic body and, 142
property rights and, 149–54
race and nationality in, 147–48
sperm donation in, 147
urine in, 148
vocabulary for, 143–44
whiteness and, 146–47

Global Egg Donors (United States), 5, 92, 108n6
global reproduction, 39, 49, 159
  bio-crossing in, 42–43
  as enactment, 161
  entanglements with, 44, 160, 161
  in feminist cultural analysis, 160
  as fluid, 160, 161
  human-animal crossings in, 43
  IVF and, 42
  local and, 44
  as metaphor, 160–61
  neoliberalism and, 41
  networks of, 159–62
  postcolonialism and, 40
  reproscapes and, 40–41
  time and space in, 50–51
  See also transnational market
gray thinking, 140
  gift markets and, 141

H

hair, 1
Have You Counted Your Eggs Today? (Copenhagen campaign), 22
  metaphor in, 25
  neoliberal body in, 23
  rhetoric in, 23–24, 26
  sperm in, 23, 24, 26
hCG hormone (human chorionic gonadotropin), 16, 48, 63, 76
  development of, 55–56
  HMG and, 56
  MvM and, 71
  weight loss industry and, 19n2, 72–73
  See also Pregnyl
heterosexuality, 27, 30–31, 71, 72, 82, 122, 157
  egg freezing and, 106, 152–53
  of oocyte providers, 91, 103
  of oocyte recipients, 98
HMG (human menopausal gonadotropin), 56, 63
home-pregnancy test, 63–65
human-animal crossings
  global reproduction and, 43
  MvM and, 66
  nationhood and, 43–44
  urine and, 65–66
  See also placentas
human chorionic gonadotropin. *See* hCG hormone
human menopausal gonadotropin. *See* HMG

I

imagined reproductive bodies, 84, 103–4, 141, 142, 155
  placentas and, 132–34
Independent Placenta Encapsulation Network (IPEN), 120–21, 127
informational bodies, 99, 100–101, 141, 142
informed consent
  as disentanglement tool, 151
  property rights and, 153–54
investment
  egg freezing as, 85–87, 97
  placenta as, 115, 129–31
  stem cell industry as, 115, 154
in vitro fertilization (IVF), 3, 96
  in Barbados, 8
  in Denmark, 11–12
  gift market for, 145
  globalization and, 42
  urine donation and, 6, 52
IPEN. *See* Independent Placenta Encapsulation Network
IVF. *See* in vitro fertilization
IVF-related pharmaceutical industry, 6, 52

J

Japan
  cosmetic spending in, 125
  egg freezing in, 10, 14
  placenta use and consumption in, 10, 14, 17, 112, 114–15, 124–25, 134
  whiteness in, 125, 126
Japan Bio Products, 6, 33, 124, 128

K
kinship, 49
blood and, 70
in feminist cultural analysis, 32
placenta and, 112–13, 131
urine donation and, 63, 69–70

L
Laqueur, Ernst, 12–13
leakiness, 159, 160
legislation
Convention on Human Rights and Biomedicine as, 13
in Denmark, 11, 19n7
LifebankUSA, 130, 131
liquidity, 2
local practices, 159
as enactment, 161
entanglements of global and, 44, 160, 161

M
maternal love, 113, 119, 122
menopause, 26, 55
HMG and, 56, 63
Menopur, 57
menstruation, 132
gendered hierarchy and, 7
metaphor and, 26
as waste, 7
Merck Sharp & Dohme (MSD), 52
metaphor
body as ecosystem, 25, 73
body as machine, 24–25
cultural contexts of, 25–26
global as, 160–61
in Have You Counted Your Eggs Today? campaign, 25
menstruation and, 26
mobility, 39–40, 44, 141
biological and biographical, 45
oocytes and, 45–47, 103
of placentas, 47–48
reproflow and, 45
technology and, 21–22
upward, 3, 125–26, 128
of urine donation, 48–49
value and, 22
mobility turn, 21, 140–41
Moeders voor Moeders (Mothers for Mothers) (MvM), 16, 48, 56
altruistic donation practice for, 54, 55, 62, 76
Aspen Oss and, 52, 54, 59
collection process by, 58–59
disgust and, 67–68
eco-friendly fertilizer of, 69
hCG and, 71
human-animal crossings at, 66
narratives of, 62–63
pharmaceutical body and, 70–71
philanthropic body and, 74
promotional material of, 53, 54, 60–62
provider criteria for, 54, 55
race and, 60, 61, 62
rhetoric of, 61
secrecy and, 68
sisterhood and, 52, 62, 76
Mol, Annemarie, 30–31
morals
bio-objectification and, 34
limits of, 2
odor and, 67
optimization and, 5
potentiality and, 7
Mothers for Mothers. *See* Moeders voor Moeders
MSD. *See* Merck Sharp & Dohme
MvM. *See* Moeders voor Moeders

N
NASA, 1
nationality
gift market and, 147–48
oocyte providers and, 91–92, 99, 148
whiteness and, 125
neocolonialism, 40
neoliberalism
entrepreneurial body and, 155–56
in feminist rhetorical and communication analysis, 23–24, 26–27

gift discourse and, 4
global reproduction and, 41
in Have You Counted Your Eggs Today? campaign, 23
individuals in, 3
placenta consumption and, 122–23, 133
Netherlands, 10–11, 14
Akzo Pharma factory in, 16
Organon Limited Company in, 13
pharmaceutical companies in, 12–13
urine donation in, 12–13, 14, 16, 48–49, 52–54
Waternet, 53
See also Aspen Oss; Merck Sharp & Dohme; Moeders voor Moeders

O

odor
moral identity and, 67
of urine, 66–68
oocyte providers
age and, 103, 104–5
in Barbados, 82–83
bland reproductive bodies of, 98–100
empowerment of, 100, 103, 105
exoticism of, 86–87, 101–3
heterosexuality of, 91, 103
imagined recipient and, 103–4
informational bodies of, 99, 100–101, 141
nationality of, 91–92, 99, 148
physical traits of, 91–92, 99–100, 102–3, 149
pride of, 105–6
race and, 91–92, 148
rightful, 103–4
separation of recipients and, 97–98
Spanish, 45, 51n5, 81–82, 101–3, 107n3, 141
whiteness and, 91
oocytes, 1–2, 32, 107n2
altruism and, 88, 89, 141, 158
assemblage ethnography of, 81–83
bio-objectification of, 34
countries and, 10, 14
distributive value of, 105–6
entanglements of, 91
entrepreneurial value of, 105–7
excess of data for, 10
in feminist affect and materialist analyses, 33, 93–94
in feminist cultural analysis, 81
as frozen assets, 17
gift and commodity framework for, 88–93
globalized femininity and, 89, 92–93, 103, 107
heterosexuality and, 91, 98, 103
intersectional power dynamics for, 148
as microcosms of self, 94–95, 97
mobility and, 45–47, 103
as "own" babies, 93, 96–97, 99, 146, 162
plentitude of, 85
price for, 1, 107n1, 149
regenerative value of, 106
reproductive intentions and, 83
reproductive path of, 97–98
Russian, 45
"simply" describing, 95
stem cell industry and, 42, 46–47, 106, 154, 156, 157
stereotypes for, 16
technology and, 33
as tiny cells, 93, 94–96, 97
transnational market for, 5, 44
waste and value of, 34, 84–88, 163
See also egg freezing
OpenBiome, 1
optimization, 5
Organon Limited Company, 13
Oudshoorn, Nelly, 55
"own" children, 93, 96–97, 99, 146, 162

P

peecycling movement, 52

PG 600, 65
pharmaceutical and cosmetics industries, 11, 14, 142
IVF-related, 6, 52
in the Netherlands, 12–13
placentas in, 5, 6, 17, 47, 111, 123–28, 134–35, 148–49, 153–54
pharmaceutical body
MvM and, 70–71
Pregnyl advertisements and, 72
weight loss and, 72–73
philanthropic body
altruism and gift giving in, 142
in feminist rhetorical and communication analysis, 23, 26–27
MvM and, 74
urine donation and, 73–74
placentas, 1–2, 32, 38, 157
assemblage of, 10
back-to-nature argument for, 121
as bioart, 115, 128–29
biobanking and, 130–31
as biocapital, 130
as biomedical evidence, 113, 115, 118–19
as cannibalism, 119–20
commodity framework for, 17
as consumable nutrients, 113
cooking shows on, 117, 118, 119
cost of encapsulated, 121
cultural and commodity meanings for, 17
Danish porcine placentas, 5, 11, 17, 21, 43, 111–12, 117, 126–27, 136n6, 136n8, 159–60
Denmark clinical practices for, 115, 116, 118, 158
empowerment and, 120, 127–28, 132–33, 154
encapsulation of, 120–22, 135, 136n16
in European Union, 112, 132–33, 137n19
in feminist affect and materialist analyses, 33
feminist cultural analysis and, 113
in feminist rhetorical and communication analysis, 118
global reproduction and, 43
human rights and, 120
imagined bodies of, 132–34
as investment, 115, 129–31
IPEN on consumption of, 120–21, 127
in Japan, 10, 14, 17, 112, 114–15, 124–25, 134
Japan Bio Products and, 6, 33, 124, 128
kinship and, 112–13, 131
as maternal love, 113, 119, 122
as matter out of place, 36
mobility of, 47–48
neoliberal maternity and, 122–23, 133
as novel food, 132–33, 137n19
pharmaceutical and cosmetics industries and, 5, 6, 17, 47, 111, 123–28, 134–35, 148–49, 153–54
physical attributes of, 110–11
placenta sites, 111–12
potentiality of, 6
regulations on, 112
as rejuvenating ingredient, 113, 115
rhetoric of, 118
ritualization practices for, 135
stem cell industry and, 112, 128, 130, 131
tales of, 112–15
tree burial of, 113, 114
in United Kingdom and United States, 10, 14, 112
upward mobility and, 125–26, 128
as waste, 113, 115–19, 134
whiteness and, 123–27, 133–34
potentiality
moral reasoning and, 7
reproductive waste and, 6
pregnancy test
feminist cultural analysis on, 64
history of, 63–64
as low-tech, 64–65

Pregnyl, 6, 54, 56, 57, 65, 76
MSD making, 52
pharmaceutical body and, 72
uses of, 52
price
of egg freezing, 108n4
of encapsulated placentas, 121
for oocytes, 1, 107n1, 149
productive bodies, 152
productive work, 156–57
property rights, 149
choice and, 152
in Findley v. Lee, 150–51
informed consent and, 153–54
productive bodies and, 152
reproductive objects without owners and, 151
Thiering and, 150
Proposition 71, 38, 51n4

R

race
colorism and, 127
Danish reproduction campaigns and, 27
gift market and, 147–48
"mix-up," 147–48
MvM and, 60, 61, 62
oocyte providers and, 91–92, 148
See also whiteness
Recycle Yourself campaign, 36
regenerative labor, 155
as active, 157
as disentanglement, 156
femininity and, 157–58
regenerative value, 106
reproductive body, 7, 105
bland, 98–100
disciplined porous body as, 74–76
entrepreneurial body as, 23, 25, 26–27, 142, 155–56, 158
exotic body as, 86–87, 101–3
fragmented, 16, 18
imagined, 84, 103–4, 132–34, 141, 142, 155
informational bodies as, 99, 100–101, 141, 142
male, 25
philanthropic body as, 23, 26–27, 73–74, 142
potential of, 4–5
rightful, 103–4
See also neoliberalism
reproductive donations. *See specific topics*
reproductive objects without owners, 151
reproductive property rights. *See* property rights
reproductive value, 17–18, 50, 158–59, 165
biovalue as, 18, 38–39
distributive, 105–6
dynamic process of, 36–37
of egg freezing, 106–7, 163
entanglements of, 38
entrepreneurial value of oocytes, 105–7
mobility and, 22
oocytes and, 34, 84–88, 105–6, 163
regenerative, 106
urine donation and, 48–49, 52, 63
reproductive waste, 2, 17–18, 50, 158–59, 162, 165–66
biocapital as, 37
biopower and, 35
disgust and, 35
dynamic process of, 36–37
egg freezing and, 85
entanglements of, 38
as matter out of place, 35–36
menstruation as, 7
oocytes and, 34, 84–88, 163
placenta as, 113, 115–19, 134
potentiality and, 6
recycling and, 36
understanding, 34–35
urine donation and, 48–49, 52, 63
reproflow, 44–45

repro-politics, 158
  leakiness in, 159
reproscapes
  fertility consumers and, 41
  global reproduction and, 40–41
  reproflow and, 45
  stratified, 41
reusability and extensibility
  autonomy and, 164
  commodification and, 148
  feminist cultural politics of, 140, 141, 159, 163–65
Rich Earth Institute, 77n3
  urine as fertilizer for, 53
rightful bodies, 103–4

S
Serono
  artificial creation by, 57
  urine donation and, 56–57
"Should I Defrost My Freezer Boys?" (Whippman), 93
Spain, 10–11, 14, 16–17
  assemblage ethnography in, 81–83
  exoticism of, 101
  as fertility hub, 12
  oocyte providers in, 45, 51n5, 81–82, 101–3, 107n3, 141
speculative value, 106–7
sperm donation, 140
  commodity market for, 144–45, 147
  gift market and, 147
  in Have You Counted Your Eggs Today? campaign, 23, 24, 26
  price of, 1
Spies. *See* Do It for Denmark and Do It for Mom
stem cell industry, 38–40, 132
  bio-crossings and, 42–43
  as investment, 115, 154
  oocytes and, 42, 46–47, 106, 154, 156, 157
  placenta in, 112, 128, 130, 131
  Proposition 71 and, 38, 51n4
stool, 1
surrogate, 1

T
Take Back Your Fertility seminar, 17, 97
Thiering, Jordan, 150
transnational feminists, 146
transnational market, 10, 33
  European Union and, 5
  fertility coordinators in, 28–29
  for oocytes, 5, 44
  urine in, 44
Traveling Donors (South Africa), 5

U
United Kingdom
  egg freezing in, 10
  IPEN of, 120–21, 127
  placenta consumption in, 10, 14, 112
  Take Back Your Fertility seminar in, 17, 97
United States
  abortion in, 7
  egg freezing in, 10, 14
  Global Egg Donors in, 5, 92, 108n6
  IVF-related pharmaceutical industry in, 6
  placenta consumption in, 10, 14, 112
  Proposition 71 in, 38, 51n4
  Rich Earth Institute in, 53, 77n3
upward mobility, 3, 125–26, 128
urine donation, 1–2, 5, 32, 157. *See also* Moeders voor Moeders
  abjection theory and, 66
  animal, 13
  artificial creation replacing, 56, 57
  assemblage of, 10
  blood donation compared to, 56–57, 60, 63
  breast milk and, 60
  countries and, 14
  demand for, 56
  disciplined porous body and, 74–76
  as eco-friendly, 68–69

entanglement of, 60
as evidence, 63–65
exclusion in, 55
feminist cultural analyses of, 3
as fertilizer, 53
gift and commodity framework for, 48–49, 59
gift market framework for, 148
hCG hormone in, 16, 19n2, 48, 55–56, 63, 71, 72–73, 76
history of, 55–59
HMG and, 56
human-animal crossings and, 65–66
IVF-related pharmaceutical industry and, 6, 52
kidneys and, 63
kinship and, 63, 69–70
maternal care and, 60–63
as medical treatment, 53, 65
menopausal urine and, 56
Menopur and, 57
mobility and, 48–49
in the Netherlands, 12–13, 14, 16, 48–49, 52–54
odor of, 66–68
peecycling movement for, 52
PG 600 and, 65
pharmaceutical body and, 70–73
philanthropic body and, 73–74
potentiality of, 6
pregnancy tests and, 63–64
as reproductive management, 65–66
Serono and, 56–57
in transnational market, 44
waste and value of, 48–49, 52, 63
Urine Therapy Association, 53, 65
uterine transplants, 4

V

value. *See* reproductive value

W

Waldby, Catherine, 38–39
waste. *See* reproductive waste
waste management labor
alienation and, 157
entrepreneurial body and, 155–56
productive work and, 156–57
regenerative labor and, 155, 156–58
Waternet, 53
welfare state, 11–12
feminist cultural politics and, 163–64
Whippman, Ruth, 93
whiteness
class and, 125–26, 128
colorism and, 127
gift market and, 146–47
in Japan, 125, 126
nationality and, 125
oocyte providers and, 91
placentas used for, 123–27, 133–34

Z

Zwanenberg, Saal van, 12–13

Fertility, Reproduction and Sexuality

GENERAL EDITORS:

Soraya Tremayne, Founding Director, Fertility and Reproduction Studies Group and Research Associate, Institute of Social and Cultural Anthropology, University of Oxford.

Marcia C. Inhorn, William K. Lanman, Jr. Professor of Anthropology and International Affairs, Yale University.

Philip Kreager, Director, Fertility and Reproduction Studies Group, and Research Associate, Institute of Social and Cultural Anthropology and Institute of Human Sciences, University of Oxford.

Volume 1
Managing Reproductive Life: Cross-Cultural Themes in Fertility and Sexuality
Edited by Soraya Tremayne

Volume 2
Modern Babylon? Prostituting Children in Thailand
Heather Montgomery

Volume 3
Reproductive Agency, Medicine and the State: Cultural Transformations in Childbearing
Edited by Maya Unnithan-Kumar

Volume 4
A New Look at Thai AIDS: Perspectives from the Margin
Graham Fordham

Volume 5
Breast Feeding and Sexuality: Behaviour, Beliefs and Taboos among the Gogo Mothers in Tanzania
Mara Mabilia

Volume 6
Ageing without Children: European and Asian Perspectives on Elderly Access to Support Networks
Edited by Philip Kreager and Elisabeth Schröder-Butterfill

Volume 7
Nameless Relations: Anonymity, Melanesia and Reproductive Gift Exchange between British Ova Donors and Recipients
Monica Konrad

Volume 8
Population, Reproduction and Fertility in Melanesia
Edited by Stanley J. Ulijaszek

Volume 9
Conceiving Kinship: Assisted Conception, Procreation and Family in Southern Europe
Monica M. E. Bonaccorso

Volume 10
Where There Is No Midwife: Birth and Loss in Rural India
Sarah Pinto

Volume 11
Reproductive Disruptions: Gender, Technology, and Biopolitics in the New Millennium
Edited by Marcia C. Inhorn

Volume 12
Reconceiving the Second Sex: Men, Masculinity, and Reproduction
Edited by Marcia C. Inhorn, Tine Tjørnhøj-Thomsen, Helene Goldberg, and Maruska la Cour Mosegaard

Volume 13
Transgressive Sex: Subversion and Control in Erotic Encounters
Edited by Hastings Donnan and Fiona Macgowan

Volume 14
European Kinship in the Age of Biotechnology
Edited by Jeanette Edwards and Carles Salazar

Volume 15
Kinship and Beyond: The Genealogical Model Reconsidered
Edited by Sandra Bamford and James Leach

Volume 16
Islam and New Kinship: Reproductive Technology and the Shariah in Lebanon
Morgan Clarke

Volume 17
Childbirth, Midwifery and Concepts of Time
Edited by Christine McCourt

Volume 18
Assisting Reproduction, Testing Genes: Global Encounters with the New Biotechnologies
Edited by Daphna Birenbaum-Carmeli and Marcia C. Inhorn

Volume 19
Kin, Gene, Community: Reproductive Technologies among Jewish Israelis
Edited by Daphna Birenbaum-Carmeli and Yoram S. Carmeli

Volume 20
Abortion in Asia: Local Dilemmas, Global Politics
Edited by Andrea Whittaker

Volume 21
Unsafe Motherhood: Mayan Maternal Mortality and Subjectivity in Post-War Guatemala
Nicole S. Berry

Volume 22
Fatness and the Maternal Body: Women's Experiences of Corporeality and the Shaping of Social Policy
Edited by Maya Unnithan-Kumar and Soraya Tremayne

Volume 23
Islam and Assisted Reproductive Technologies: Sunni and Shia Perspectives
Edited by Marcia C. Inhorn and Soraya Tremayne

Volume 24
Militant Lactivism? Attachment Parenting and Intensive Motherhood in the UK and France
Charlotte Faircloth

Volume 25
Pregnancy in Practice: Expectation and Experience in the Contemporary US
Sallie Han

Volume 26
Nighttime Breastfeeding: An American Cultural Dilemma
Cecília Tomori

Volume 27
Globalized Fatherhood
Edited by Marcia C. Inhorn, Wendy Chavkin, and José-Alberto Navarro

Volume 28
Cousin Marriages: Between Tradition, Genetic Risk and Cultural Change
Edited by Alison Shaw and Aviad Raz

Volume 29
Achieving Procreation: Childlessness and IVF in Turkey
Merve Demircioğlu Göknar

Volume 30
Thai *in Vitro*: Gender, Culture and Assisted Reproduction
Andrea Whittaker

Volume 31
Assisted Reproductive Technologies in the Third Phase: Global Encounters and Emerging Moral Worlds
Edited by Kate Hampshire and Bob Simpson

Volume 32
Parenthood between Generations: Transforming Reproductive Cultures
Edited by Siân Pooley and Kaveri Qureshi

Volume 33
Patient-Centred IVF: Bioethics and Care in a Dutch Clinic
Trudie Gerrits

Volume 34
Conceptions: Infertilities and Procreative Technologies in India
Aditya Bharadwaj

Volume 35
The Online World of Surrogacy
Zsuzsa Berend

Volume 36
Fertility, Conjuncture, Difference: Anthropological Approaches to the Heterogeneity of Modern Fertility Declines
Edited by Philip Kreager and Astrid Bochow

Volume 37
The Anthropology of the Fetus
Edited by Sallie Han, Tracy K. Betsinger, and Amy K. Scott

Volume 38
Reconceiving Muslim Men: Love and Marriage, Family and Care in Precarious Times
Edited by Marcia C. Inhorn and Nefissa Naguib

Volume 39
Global Fluids: The Cultural Politics of Reproductive Waste and Value
Charlotte Kroløkke